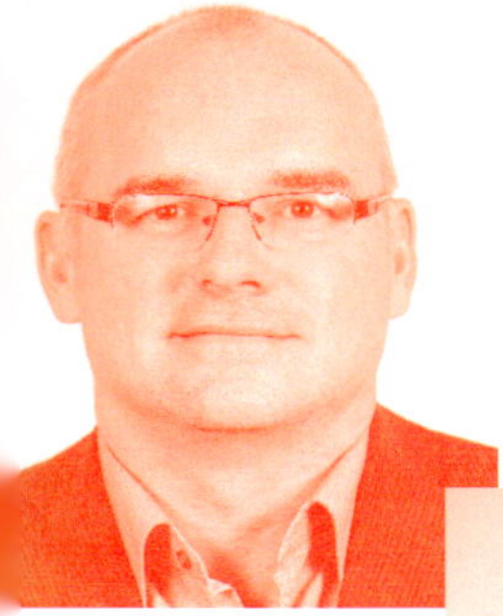
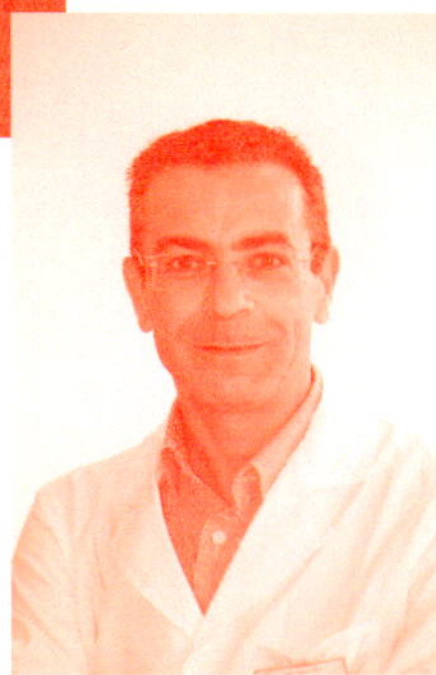
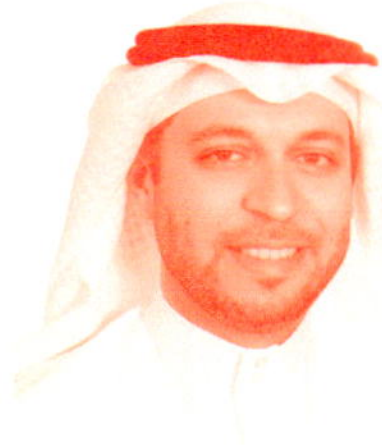
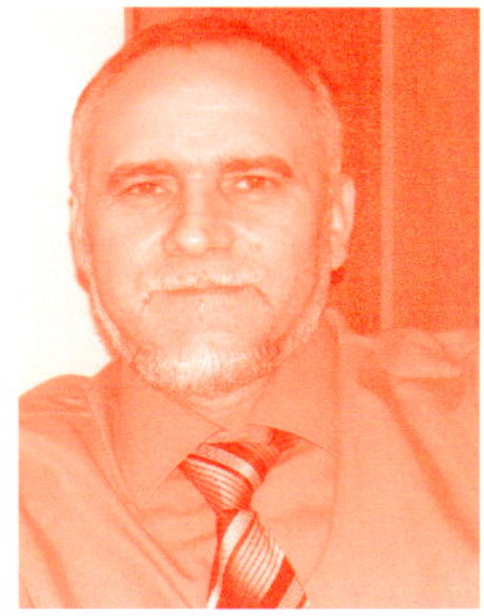
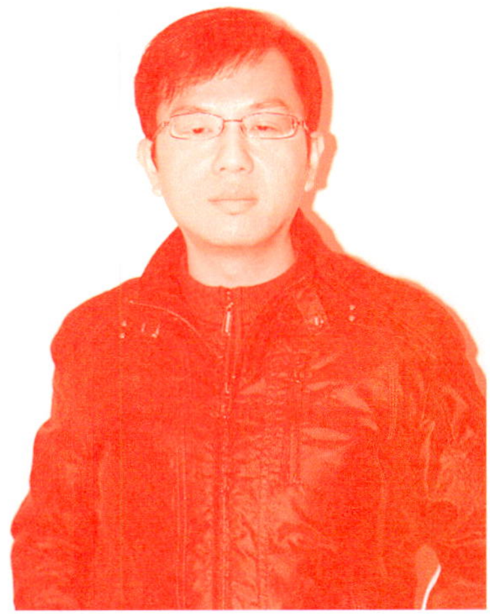
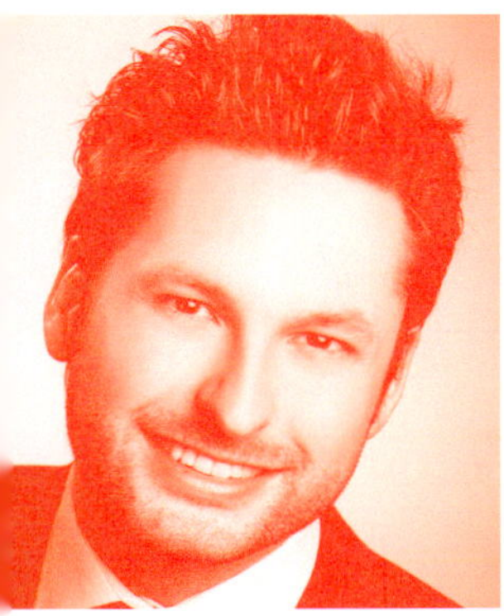
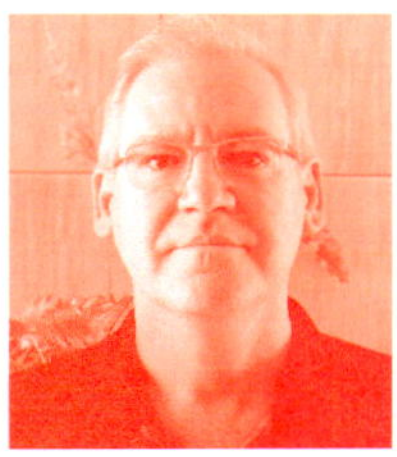

IntechOpen

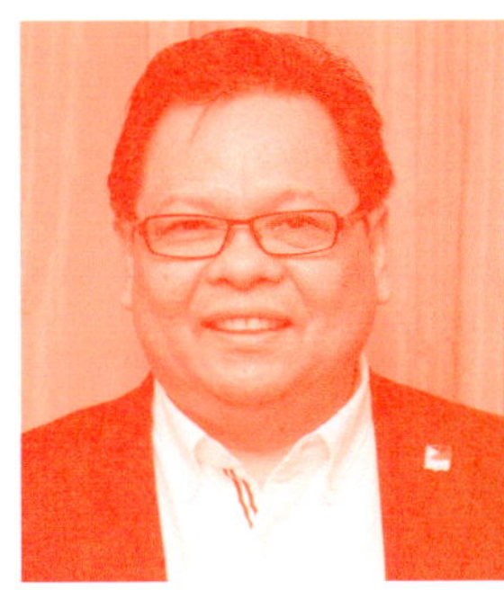
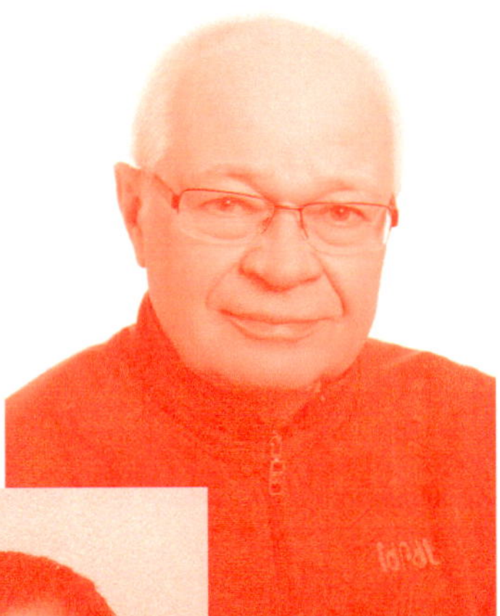
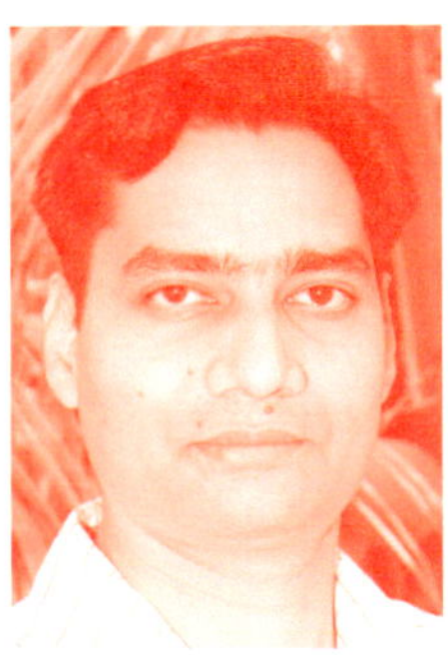
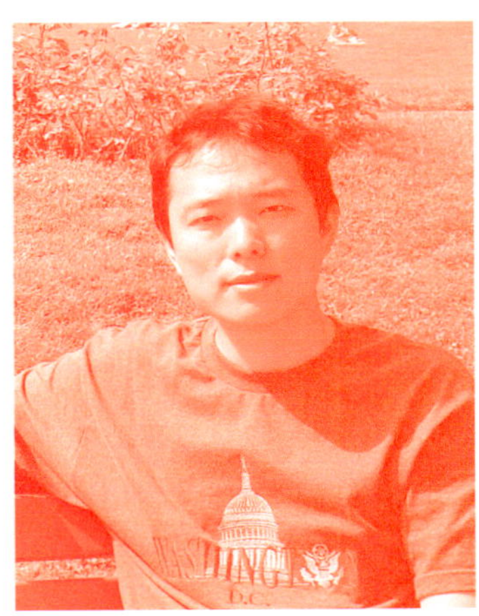
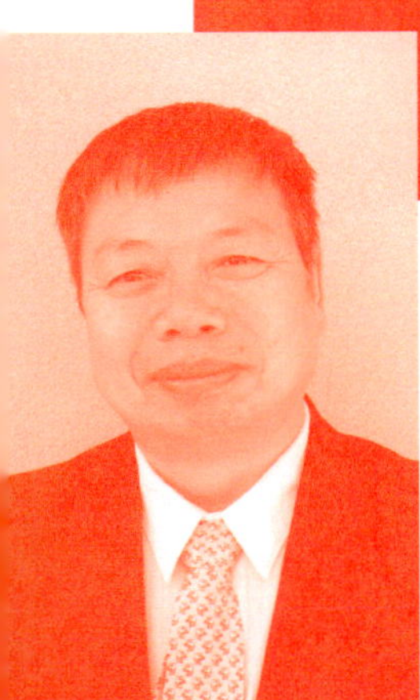
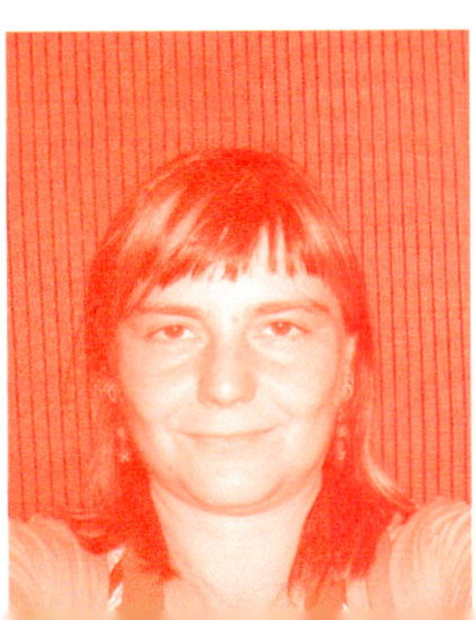

New Insight into Brucella Infection and Foodborne Diseases

Edited by Mitra Ranjbar,
Marzieh Nojomi and Maria T. Mascellino

Published in London, United Kingdom

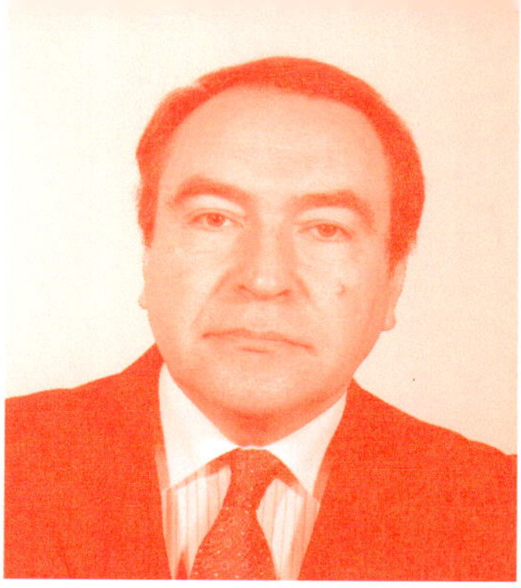
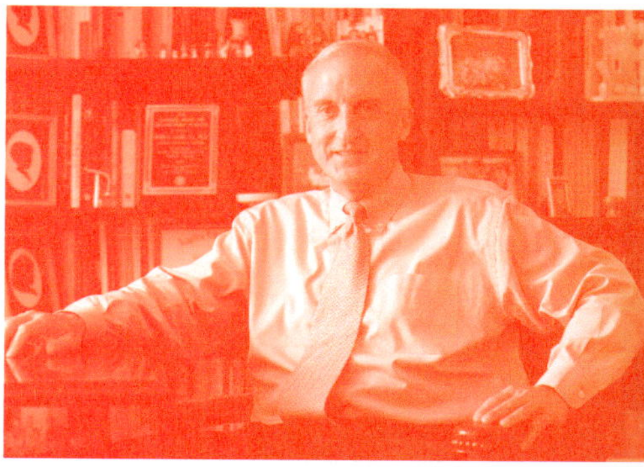
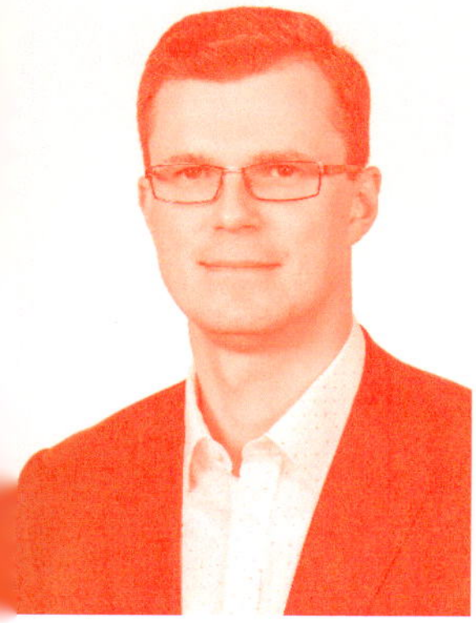
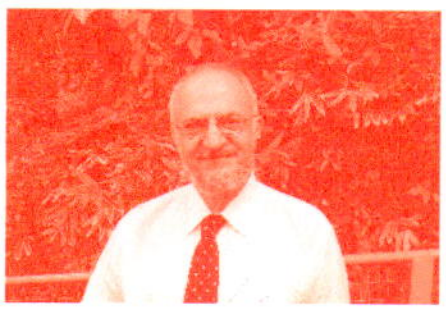
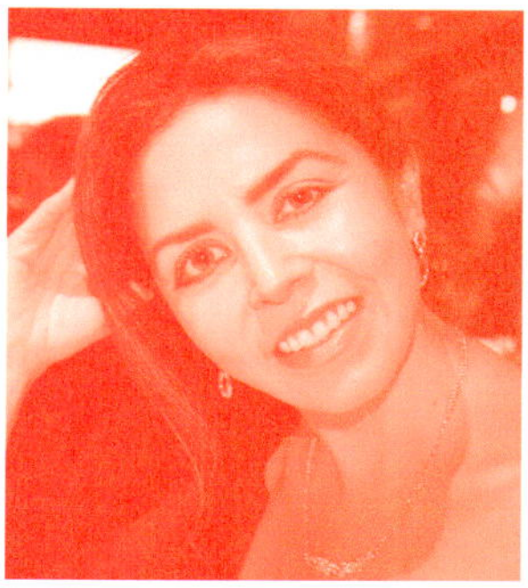

Supporting open minds since 2005

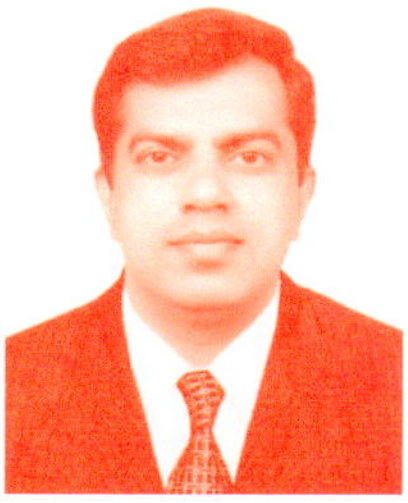
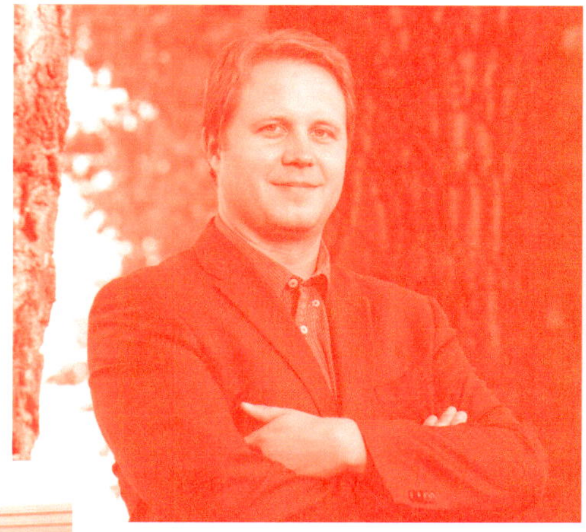
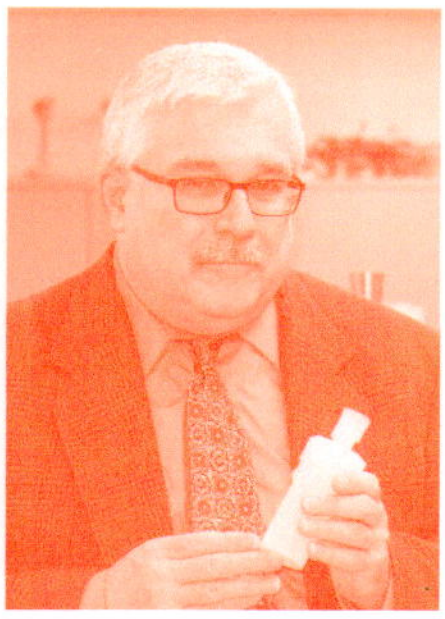
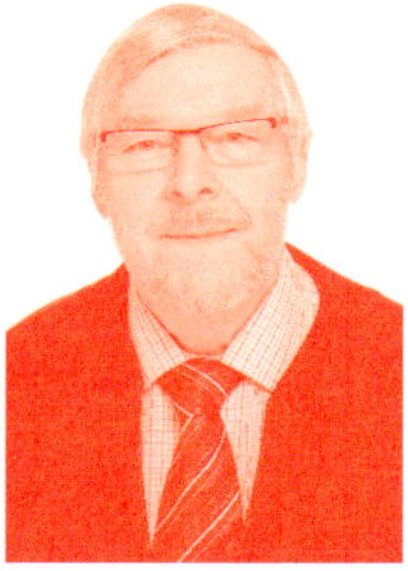
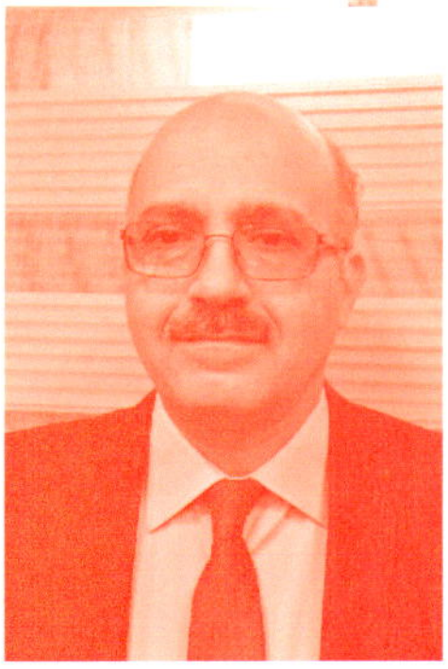
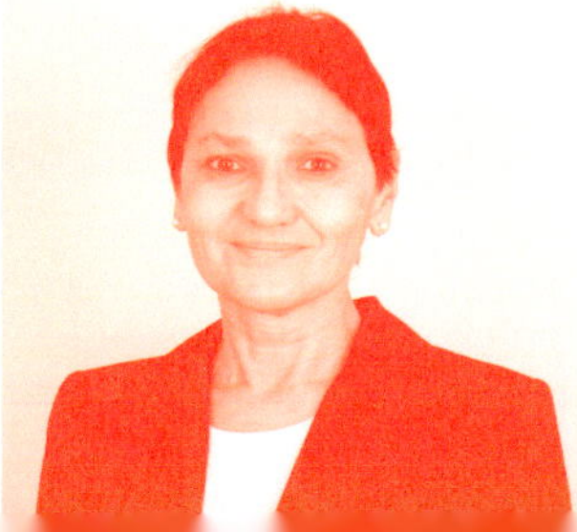
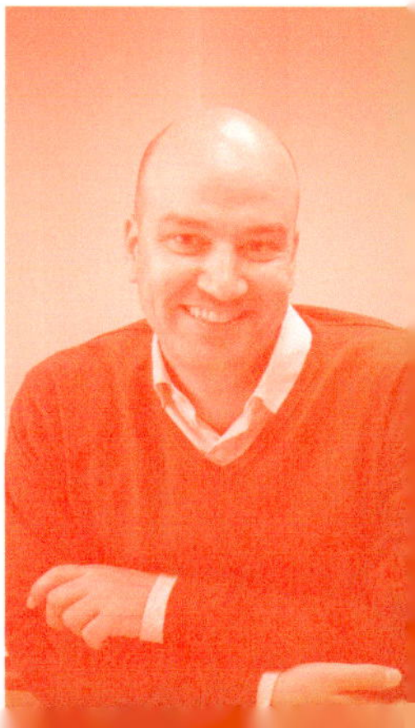

New Insight into Brucella Infection and Foodborne Diseases
http://dx.doi.org/10.5772/intechopen.77695
Edited by Mitra Ranjbar, Marzieh Nojomi and Maria T. Mascellino

Contributors
Mashooq Dar, Peerzada Tajamul Mumtaz, Shakil Ahmad Bhat, Qamar Taban, Syed Mudasir Ahmad, Nur Aziemah Abd Rashid, Ismail Abustan, Dilek Çam, Burton Blais, Catherine Carrillo, Adam Koziol, Neil Vary, Aneela Durrani, Muhammad Usman, Zain Kazmi, Muhaamd Husnain, Sara Arias, Julio C. Garcia, Baldomero Molina, David I Martinez Herrera, Violeta Pardío, Ricardo Flores Castro, Jose Francisco Morales Alvarez, Jose Alfredo Villagomez Cortes, Fatemeh Eghbalian, Shokoufeh Savaj, Maria Teresa Mascellino

First published in London, United Kingdom, 2020 by IntechOpen
IntechOpen is the global imprint of INTECHOPEN LIMITED, registered in England and Wales, registration number: 11086078, 7th floor, 10 Lower Thames Street, London, EC3R 6AF, United Kingdom
Printed in Croatia

British Library Cataloguing-in-Publication Data
A catalogue record for this book is available from the British Library

Additional hard and PDF copies can be obtained from orders@intechopen.com

New Insight into Brucella Infection and Foodborne Diseases
Edited by Mitra Ranjbar, Marzieh Nojomi and Maria T. Mascellino
p. cm.
Print ISBN 978-1-78985-097-0
Online ISBN 978-1-78985-098-7
eBook (PDF) ISBN 978-1-83962-778-1

For EU product safety concerns:
IN TECH d.o.o., Prolaz Marije Krucifikse Kozulić 3, 51000 Rijeka, Croatia, info@intechopen.com or visit our website at intechopen.com.

Meet the editors

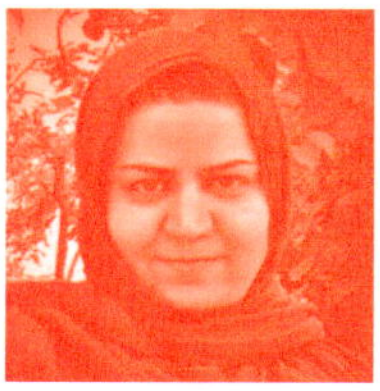

Professor Mitra Ranjbar, MD, specializes in infectious diseases and tropical medicine as well as a course of MPH. She has worked for about 20 years as a university teacher and investigator. The majority of her work and research is about brucellosis (clinical trials and complications of brucellosis such as neurobrucellosis, osteoarticular brucellosis, immunology of brucellosis) and endemic infectious diseases in Iran such as typhoid fever, cholera, viral hepatitis, etc. She has written more than 60 papers about infectious diseases. Dr. Mitra Ranjbar is the Dean of the Department of Infectious Diseases at the Iran University of Medical Sciences, Tehran, Iran.

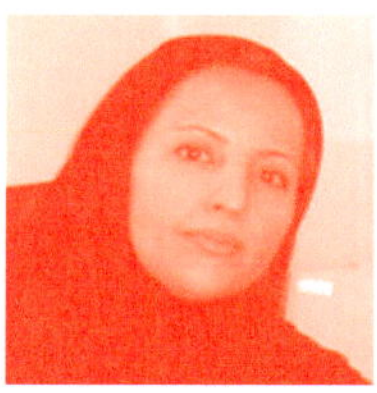

Professor Marzieh Nojomi, MD, MPH, is specialized in community and preventive medicine as well as flow of clinical epidemiology. She has worked for 20 years as a university teacher and investigator. The majority of her work and research is about public and community health. Dr. Nojomi has written more than two hundred papers about community medicine, women's health, and epidemiology of disease. Dr. Nojomi is the dean of the Department of Community and Family Medicine and also the head of Preventive Medicine and Public Health Research Center at Iran University of Medical Sciences, Tehran, Iran.

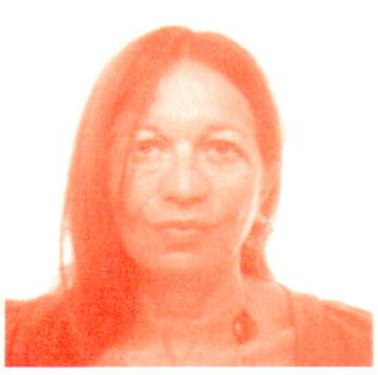

Maria T. Mascellino has completed her MD at the age of 25 years in Rome during the period of 1980 and specialization in Clinical Microbiology from Sapienza University of Rome (Italy). She works as aggregate professor in the Department of Public Health and Infectious Diseases. She has published other than 100 papers in reputed journals and has been serving as an editorial board member of repute. She is editor of the book "Bacterial and Mycotic infections in immune-compromised hosts" (OMICS group) and of the book "Salmonella: a re-emerging pathogen" (InTech). She is a reviewer for important scientific international Journals and Research Projects from Ministry of University. She has attended national and international Conferences as speaker presenting relevant research topics.

Contents

Preface

Brucellosis is a major zoonotic disease. Elimination of human disease depends on the prevention and control of animal infections. In endemic settings, brucellosis typically affects rural communities with inadequate access to healthcare and preventative education. There is often a history of illness in the family, occupational exposure, or travel from an endemic area.

The clinical features are variable, most commonly presenting as nonspecific fever, accompanied by musculoskeletal pain in almost half of the patients. The most important differential diagnosis is tuberculosis, especially in localized infections. Less common manifestations include prostatitis, cystitis, interstitial nephritis, or glomerulonephritis. Infection among children is generally more benign than in adults with respect to likelihood and severity of complications and response to treatment. Brucellosis in pregnancy is associated with the risk of spontaneous abortion, premature delivery, miscarriage, and intrauterine infection with fetal death. The diagnosis should be confirmed by culture of blood or other sterile fluids, e.g. joint aspirates or by serological tests.

The microbiology laboratory should be warned if brucellosis is suspected, both to optimize testing strategies and to reduce the significant risk of laboratory-acquired infection. Treatment regimens should include at least two antimicrobial agents for at least 6 weeks, in order to prevent relapse. Aminoglycoside-containing regimens are superior. More prolonged treatment with a triple antimicrobial combination may be required for complicated infections.

The approach taken by the authors in this book is resolutely practical as they have tried to introduce and discuss therapeutic trials in cattle, the *brucella* spp. vaccines and their possible implications to control programs, molecular targets, and methods for differentiation of species and biovars. In addition, the latest updates of antibiotic therapy of brucellosis are described, which makes the book easier to consult. Kidney involvement in brucellosis and neonatal brucellosis are included in this book.

This book is the result of several months of outstanding efforts by authors and revision of the content by experts in the field of brucellosis. This book is a valid resource and is intended for everyone interested in infectious disease to learn the most important aspects of brucellosis.

Please do not hesitate to share with us your invaluable comments to improve the next editions. We are deeply appreciative of our colleagues as this work would not have been possible without their contribution.

Mitra Ranjbar, MD
Professor of Infectious Diseases,
Department of Infectious Diseases,
Iran University of Medical Sciences,
Tehran, Iran

Maria T. Mascellino
Department of Public Health and Infectious Diseases,
Sapienza University of Rome,
Rome, Italy

Marzieh Nojomi
Iran University of Medical Sciences,
Tehran, Iran

Chapter 1

Evaluation of Therapeutic Trials in Bovines

Aneela Zameer Durrani, Muhammad Usman, Zain Kazmi and Muhammad Husnain

Abstract

Brucellosis is one of the most common and economically important zoonotic diseases globally. Office International des Epizooties (OIE) listed it as the second most important zoonotic disease. The disease affects almost all animals but importantly buffalo. The disease manifests itself in the form of abortion, still births, weak calves, infertility, and specific lesions on reproductive organs. It is prevalent worldwide but still a neglected disease. As a zoonotic disease its importance is multifarious for animals as well as public health. Taking into account poor health facilities and unawareness, its control becomes very significant. The difficulty to treat this disease and its zoonotic potential compel slaughtering as a best strategy to get rid of this disease. There are not too many therapeutic trials conducted to control bovine brucellosis. Instead many therapeutic trials have been conducted for treating human brucellosis. The therapeutic trial requires long term administration of drugs (almost 6 weeks) without any surety of complete recovery so it is a preferred practice to eradicate the animal or sell it out instead of treating.

Keywords: *Brucella*, bovines, therapeutic trial, slaughtering, zoonotic

1. Introduction

Brucellosis is one of the most common and economically important zoonotic diseases globally [1]. It was first discovered by Bruce in 1887. It is also known as undulant fever, Mediterranean fever, Epizootic abortion, Enzootic abortion, Malta fever, and Bang's disease [2, 3]. It is considered as the most rapidly spreading disease by the World Health Organization (WHO), Food and Agriculture Organization (FAO), and Office International des Epizooties (OIE) [4]. Significant economic losses due to brucellosis are abortion, low milk yield, low conception rate and culling of animal [5]. Central Asia, the Middle East and adjacent subtropical geographies are among those with the highest incidence of brucellosis among humans and livestock worldwide [6]. There is a reason to believe that the burden caused by brucellosis in low-income countries in Asia and Africa is large [1]. Important animal species that can get this disease include cattle, buffalo, swine, sheep, goats, camels, dogs and being zoonotic can also infect humans [7]. Prevalence of brucellosis in Buffalo is 5.05% in Pakistan [8]. This is suggested by quite an old study and conduction of a new research is required to study the current trends of brucellosis in Pakistan. It is for sure that its prevalence has increased to threatening level.

Brucella is Gram-negative, nonmotile, coccobacilli or small rods intracellular pathogen that are taxonomically categorized in the in the class α-proteobacteria, order

Rhizobiales, family Brucellaceae. It is caused by ingestion of unpasteurized milk or undercooked meat from infected animals, or close contact with their secretions [3]. It is caused by different bacteria of the genus *Brucella* characterized by abortion epididymis and orchitus. Brucellosis causes abortions in the third trimester of pregnancy when unvaccinated cattle are exposed to the infectious organism. Brucellosis has been reported since long in Pakistan and due to its increasing prevalence emphasis has been put on regular screening of livestock herds and of animals brought at abattoirs and at livestock markets [9]. The overall prevalence of brucellosis in Punjab is found to be 2.5%.

2. Diagnosis of brucellosis

Brucella spp. is considered as the most common laboratory-acquired pathogens. Several serological tests have been widely used for diagnosis of *Brucella* such are Rose Bengal plate test (RBPT), standard tube agglutination test (STAT), complement fixation test (CFT), enzyme linked immunosorbant assay (ELISA). Besides these, polymerase chain reaction (PCR)-based identification and typing and fluorescence polarization assays (FPA) are also important diagnostic tools [10]. These all diagnostic tools have been employed by various researchers to find out brucellosis. Shafee and other in 2011 used MRT and i-ELISA to find out overall prevalence of brucellosis in Quetta, capital of Baluchistan province of Pakistan [11].

ELISA and PCR are more specific tests to diagnose brucellosis but there are various limitations to these tests. Both of these tests are expansive and need sophisticated equipment to perform. Both cannot be performed in field conditions.

2.1 Therapeutic trial of brucellosis

The bovine brucellosis is very prevalent but a neglected disease on the whole. The countries which are declared as *Brucella* free countries managed to attain this status through slaughtering and destroying the *Brucella* positive animals along with effective vaccination. The literature confirmed that no country overcome it through treating the *Brucella* positive animals. The main reason behind this practice is the long duration of therapeutic trial, i.e., almost 6 weeks without any surety of complete recovery. In most of the cases, animals relapse the disease or act as a carrier for rest of their life.

Alavi and Ali Reza treated *Brucella* positive patients with doxycycline-rifampin and doxycycline-cortimoxazol and compared their efficacy. They concluded that the later combination has a better efficacy than former [12]. In another study the therapeutic efficacy of doxycycline and rifampicin (DR) with a doxycycline plus streptomycin (DS) were compared. It was concluded that doxycycline-aminoglycoside combination has a better efficacy and doxycycline-rifampin and doxycycline-cotrimoxazole should be the alternative regimens [10].

Hari and Sughanda conducted a different type of research and checked immunotherapeutic response in cattle using a specific biomarker. They are against brucellosis. The SL induced strong antibody response and RL reported successful use of phage lysates of RB51 (RL) and S19 (SL) against brucellosis. The SL induced strong antibody response and RL stimulated cell mediated immunity (CMI). Other than these, no therapeutic trial are available in literature for evaluation. The reasons of which have already been discussed.

3. Conclusions

Although bovine brucellosis is very prevalent and now reemerging still no therapeutic trial has been conducted since now. The main reasons behind include the complex nature of *Brucella* infection, long duration of therapy, and relapse of disease after treatment.

Acknowledgements

This chapter is supported by PAK US Science and Technology project entitled "Capacity building for vector born neglected diseases in livestock."

Conflict of interest

The authors declare that there is no conflict of interest regarding the use of this data.

Abbreviations

OIE	Office International des Epizooties
WHO	World Health Organization
FAO	Food and Agriculture Organization
FPA	fluorescence polarization assays
CMI	cell mediated immunity
RBPT	Rose Bengal plate test
STAT	standard tube agglutination test
CFT	complement fixation test
ELISA	enzyme linked immunosorbant assay
PCR	polymerase chain reaction

Author details

Aneela Zameer Durrani*, Muhammad Usman, Zain Kazmi and Muhammad Husnain
University of Veterinary and Animal Sciences, Lahore, Pakistan

*Address all correspondence to: aneela@uvas.edu.pk

References

[1] Godfroid J, Nielsen K, Saegerman C. Croatian Medical Journal. 2010;**51**: 296-305

[2] Abubakar M, Mansoor M, Arshad MJ. Bovine brucellosis: Old and new concepts with Pakistan perspective. Pakistan Veterinary Journal. 2012;**32**(2):147-155

[3] Bano Y, Lone SA. Brucellosis: An economically important infection. Journal of Medical Microbiology & Diagnosis. 2015;**4**:208. DOI: 10.4172/2161-0703.1000208

[4] Pappas G. The changing *Brucella* ecology: Novel reservoirs, new threats. International Journal of Antimicrobial Agents. 2010. DOI: 10.1016/j.ijantimicag.2010.06.013

[5] Gul ST, Khan A. Epidemiology and epizootology of brucellosis: A review. Pakistan Veterinary Journal. 2007;**27**(3):145-151

[6] McDermott J, Grace D, Zinsstag J. Economics of brucellosis impact and control in low-income countries. Revue scientifique et technique (International Office of Epizootics). 2013;**32**:249-261

[7] Falade S. Serological response of sheep to *Brucella* melitensis rev. 1 Vaccine. Zoonoses and Public Health. 1983;**30**(1-10):546-551

[8] Ahmad R, Munir MA. Epidemiological investigation of brucellosis in Pakistan. Pakistan Veterinary Journal. 1995;**15**:169-172

[9] Ahmad T, Iahtasham K, Saddaf R, Saeed HK, Raheela A. Prevalence of bovine brucellosis in Islamabad and Rawalpindi districts of Pakistan. Pakistan Journal of Zoology. 2016;**49**(3):761-1149. DOI: 10.17582/journal.pjz/2017.49.3.sc5

[10] Alavi SM, Alavi L. Treatment of brucellosis: A systematic review of studies in recent twenty years. Caspian Journal of Internal Medicine. 2013;**4**(2):636-641

[11] Rajala EL, Cecilia G, Isabel L, Nosirjon S, Sofia B, Ulf M. Prevalence and risk factors for *Brucella* seropositivity among sheep and goats in a peri-urban region of Tajikistan. 2016;**48**(3):553-558

[12] Alavi SM, Rajabzadeh AR. Comparison of two chemotherapy regimen: Doxycycline-rifampicin and doxycycline cotrimoxazol in the brucellosis patients AHVAZ, IRAN, 2004-2006. Pakistan Journal of Medical Sciences. 2007 (Part-II);**23**(6):889-892

Chapter 2

Comparative Field Trial Effect of *Brucella* spp. Vaccines on Seroconversion in Goats and Their Possible Implications to Control Programs

Baldomero Molina-Sánchez, David I. Martínez-Herrera, Violeta T. Pardío-Sedas, Ricardo Flores-Castro, José F. Morales-Álvarez and José A. Villagómez-Cortés

Abstract

The aim of this study was to determine the seroprevalence of *Brucella* spp. in a goat flock and the seroconversion of three groups of animals vaccinated with Rev-1 (*Brucella melitensis*), RB51, and RB51-SOD (*Brucella abortus*) to estimate the level of protection conferred on susceptible females. Seventy-two animals were used by group. Goats were older than 3 months, seronegative to brucellosis, not vaccinated previously, and kept within positive flocks. Vaccinated animals received 2 mL of product subcutaneously in the neck region. The first block was injected with Rev-1; the second received RB51, and the third group was injected with RB51-SOD. Follow-up sampling was performed at 30, 60, 90, and 365 days post-vaccination. The general prevalence of brucellosis for the three groups was 1.2% (95%CI:0.5–2.7). The seroconversion rate by day 30 after vaccination was 77.7% (95%CI:61.9–88.2) for goats vaccinated with Rev-1. At 365 days post vaccination, the percentage of seropositive goats declined to 13.8% (95%CI:6.0–28.6). At day 365 after vaccination, 2.7% (95%CI:0.4–14.1) and 5.5% (95%CI:1.5–18.1) of animals vaccinated with RB51 and RB51-SOD, respectively, became positive. Results show that the seroconversion induced by Brucella abortus RB51 and RB51-SOD vaccines is lower than that by *Brucella melitensis* Rev-1.

Keywords: *Brucella*, vaccine, seroprevalence, seroconversion, goat

1. Introduction

The brucellosis is a highly contagious disease and one of the zoonoses worldwide; most importantly, it is caused by bacteria of the genus *Brucella* [1]. This has been classified by the World Health Organization (WHO) as one of the "top 10" neglected zoonoses, a group of diseases that are simultaneously ongoing threats to human health and a source of perpetuation for poverty [2]. The importance of the disease is enormous but remains under-prioritized worldwide, especially among the pastoralists and small-scale livestock farmers. The humans can be infected by ingestion of food products such as unpasteurized milk and their derivative products contaminated with the pathogen or by direct interaction with an infected animal or by aerosol inhalation [1, 3].

In small ruminants, the brucellosis is caused by *B. melitensis* [4, 5], the most important agent that induces the disease in humans [6, 7]. The disease often occurs in cattle, sheep, and goat production units; the latter is the most important given its potential role in conveying disease to human. Because brucellosis is a public health problem, its presence and disease control strategies implemented in domestic ruminants affect the occurrence of disease in humans [8, 9]. In small ruminants, the disease is clinically characterized by a decrease in milk production, abortion, loss of weight, fetal death, placental retention, weak offspring, and acute orchitis. In dairy animals, *Brucella* spp. replicates in the mammary gland and supra-mammary lymph nodes, and infected animals continually excrete the pathogen into milk throughout their lives [10, 11].

In underdeveloped countries, vaccination is the main tool used in the control of this disease [12, 13], in particular as a preventive measure in small ruminants, and is considered necessary given the economic and medical consequences of having brucellosis in animals and people infected [14]. The main indicator of brucellosis reduction in animals is a concomitant reduction of human cases [13, 15]. In endemic areas, intensive vaccination with *B. melitensis* Rev. 1 strain in adult and young females has been developed, being the most popular vaccine for the control of brucellosis in small ruminants. The use of a reduced dose rate decreases the presence of vaccine-associated undesirable events, such as postvaccine reactors to conventional tests, abortion, and milk shedding [16]. The vaccination is recommended prior to the first gestation between 3 and 7 months of age to avoid abortion in pregnant animals [17]. When used at a reduced dose, Rev. 1 has shown to protect goats for at least 5 years after vaccination [13, 15]. El Idrissi et al. show that after vaccination, the animals vaccinated with Rev. 1 became positive to rose bengal plate test (RBPT) and complement fixation test (CFT) at 2 weeks, reaching the highest number of seroconverted animals' highest level between 2 and 6 weeks. Thereafter, the percentage of seropositive ewes declined to zero at 14 weeks after challenge. More than 75% of animals were seroconverted 15 days after challenge inoculation [18]. The seroconversion of vaccine is the persistent serological reaction, especially when animals are vaccinated as adults. These persistent serological reactions are mainly against the antigenic O-chain of the lipopolysaccharide present in smooth *Brucella* [19]. Some strains may generate diagnostic interferences in serological test [19, 20], like vaccines containing *Brucella* LPS O antigens that are detected by traditional serodiagnostic tests for brucellosis [21]. It has been reported that the average time from inoculation to seroconversion may range from 2 to 3 weeks in *B. melitensis*-infected goats, from 2 to 4 weeks in *B. abortus*-infected goats, and 3 weeks for the majority of tests evaluated with goats infected with either *Brucella* species [5, 19].

In Mexico, the vaccine RB51 was approved since 1998 as the official one for use in cattle females. The strain has been evaluated in both goat and sheep under controlled conditions with good protection against the experimental challenge with *B. melitensis*, even though protection is lower than that obtained with the Rev. 1 vaccine. Under experimental conditions no abortion occurs. Also, no postvaccination antibodies can be detected by conventional serology. The same findings have been reported after mass goat vaccination with RB51 in Veracruz, Mexico [13, 15].

Nowadays, the homologous overexpression to induce a greater and more effective immune response for the improvement of protective immunity of the vaccines has been developed. This can be achieved by introducing a plasmid within the RB51 strain with the gene that encodes the antigen expressed, along with appropriate promoters. In mouse (*Balb/c*) it has been shown that the overexpression of Cu/Zn superoxide dismutase (SOD) induces the best protection facing the experimental infection by *B. abortus* indicating that the homologous overexpression can produce a better vaccine RB51 (RB51-SOD) with an equal or better protection than that induced by Rev. 1, against the infection with *B. melitensis* [14, 19, 20]. However, there are no reports in domestic animals on the seroconversion and the vaccine efficacy. Therefore, the aim of this study was to determine the prevalence of *Brucella melitensis* in a goat flock and the seroconversion in animals vaccinated with Rev. 1 *Brucella melitensis*, RB51, and RB51-SOD *Brucella abortus* strains to estimate the level of protection conferred on susceptible females.

2. Material and methods

2.1 Study design

A phase III field trial was performed from September to December 2016 in order to determine the seroprevalence and seroconversion of goat flocks positive to brucellosis in the Xaltepec community municipality of Perote, Veracruz, Mexico, and to evaluate the protection conferred by vaccines with Rev. 1 *Brucella melitensis*, RB51, and RB51-SOD *Brucella abortus* strains.

2.2 Experimental design

The experiment was performed in two stages. In the first one, 546 animals from 14 herds with similar management, grazing, feeding, and confinement conditions were used to determine the prevalence of goat brucellosis in Xaltepec. In the second stage, groups required for vaccine evaluation were integrated by randomly selecting animals negative to serological tests meeting the inclusion criteria. Positive animals remained in the herds under field conditions in order to function as a challenge for healthy and vaccinated animals.

Sample size was calculated using Win Episcope Version 2.0 for simple random sampling, considering the 0.52% prevalence in goats reported in Veracruz by Román-Ramírez et al. of [12], a confidence interval of 95%, and an error margin of 5%. Since each animal had an identification number on its metallic earring, females were randomly assigned to each group and subgroup. For each group, the minimal calculated sample was 72 animals; each group was integrated by a vaccinated subgroup (36) and a not vaccinated or control subgroup (36). Studied groups were integrated by goats older than 3 months, seronegative to brucellosis, and not vaccinated previously and kept within positive flocks. Animals were randomly split into three groups and kept together 8 months in the flock to maintain exposure to *Brucella* spp.

2.3 Vaccination of animals

Animals in each vaccinated group received 2 mL of vaccine subcutaneously applied in the neck region. The first group was injected with Rev. 1 (*Brucella melitensis*) strain with a concentration of 1–2 × 10^9 CFU/mL, the second received RB51 strain (*Brucella abortus*) 3 × 10^8 to 3 × 10^9 CFU/mL, and the third one was injected with RB51-SOD (*Brucella abortus*) with a concentration of 3 × 10^8 to 3 × 10^9 CFU/mL. Each group had a control subgroup of unvaccinated animals which received 2 mL of PSS by subcutaneous injection in the neck region.

2.4 Sample collection

Follow-up sampling was performed at 30, 60, 90, and 365 days post vaccination by blood sampling collected from the jugular vein in vacutainer tubes without anti-coagulant (BD Vacutate, Oxford, UK). Each tube was identified with the number in the animal earring. Tubes containing blood samples were placed in a tilt position about 2 hours at room temperature allowing the separation of serum from the blood package. Later, tubes were placed into coolers at 4°C and transported to the laboratory and then were centrifuged at 1000 × *g* 10 minutes at room temperature. Finally, the serum was stored in sterile vials at −20°C until analysis.

2.5 Serological testing

Serum samples were analyzed by series using the following tests: 3% RBPT as screening and simple radial immunodifusion test (SRD) as confirmatory [5, 22].

RBPT was used as a screening test on the serum samples collected for the presence of *Brucella* agglutinins. Equal volumes of test serum and B. *abortus* antigen strain 1119-3 at 3% and pH of 3.6 (Aba Test Tarjeta 3%) (National Producer of Veterinary Biologics PRONABIVE) were added and mixed. This test has shown 98% sensitivity and 100% specificity. This test gives presumptive results.

SRD was used as a confirmatory test, and the antigen was used at a concentration of 1 mg/mL on agarose gel prepared with a glycine buffer solution and native hapten obtained from *B. melitensis* 16 M strain (produced at CENID Microbiology Animal, INIFAP). The test has shown 96% sensitivity and 80–100% specificity for the differential diagnosis between goats infected with *Brucella* spp. and those vaccinated with the Rev. 1 strain.

2.6 Analyses of data

Seroconversion produced during the observation period was calculated. Differences between groups and the significance of association were calculated by chi square (Xi^2), and the degree of association was estimated using relative risk (RR) [23]. In those cases that frequency of positive animals to tests was 0.0%, confidence interval was calculated according to Campbell et al. [24].

3. Results

The results of initial seroprevalence of brucellosis in goat flocks at Xaltepec are shown in **Tables 1** and **2**. The seroprevalence in the three groups determined by the 3% RBPT as presumptive test resulted in 22.1, 26.1, and 16.0% (95%CI: 16.5–28.9, 19.9–33.2, and 11.1–22.3, respectively).

The serum positive goats were confirmed with SRD, and the prevalence reduced to 0.5, 1.1, and 2.2% (95%CI: 0.3–3.4, 0.1–4.3, and 0.7–5.9, respectively). Thus, a general prevalence of 1.2% (95%CI: 0.5–2.7) was observed.

Tables 3–6 show the seroconversion rate in goats vaccinated with *Brucella* strain determined by RBPT at 30, 60, 90, and 365 days after vaccination. At 30 days after vaccination, the 77.7% (95%CI: 61.9–88.2) of goats vaccinated with Rev. 1 strain became positive to RBPT. Thereafter, 60 and 90 days post vaccination the percentage of seropositive goats declined to 72.2% (95%CI: 56.0–84.1) and 63.8% (95%CI: 47.5–77.5), respectively. At 365 days, 13.8% of vaccinated animals remained as seropositive to RBPT. Only two animals vaccinated with RB51 and RB5-SOD, respectively, were positive to RBPT at 30, 60, and 90 days after vaccination with

Strain	Sample size	RBPT		
		Positive	Seroprevalence (%)	95%CI
Rev. 1	185	41	22.1	16.5–28.9
RB51	180	47	26.1	19.9–33.2
RB51-SOD	181	29	16.0	11.1–22.3
Total	**546**	**117**	**21.4**	**18.1–25.1**

Table 1.
Seroprevalence of brucellosis rate by RBPT in goat flocks of Xaltepec municipality Perote, Veracruz, Mexico.

Strain	Sample size	SRD		
		Positive	Seroprevalence (%)	95%CI
Rev. 1	41	1	0.5	0.3–3.4
RB51	47	2	1.1	0.1–4.3
RB51-SOD	29	4	2.2	0.7–5.9
Total	**117**	7	**1.2**	**0.5–2.7**

Table 2.
Seroprevalence of brucellosis rate by SRD in goat flocks of Xaltepec municipality Perote, Veracruz, Mexico.

Group/subgroup		N	Time after vaccination (days)		
			30		
			Positive	Seroconversion rate (%)	95%CI
Rev 1	Vaccinated	36	28 a	77.7	61.9–88.2
	Control	36	4 b	11.1	4.4–25.3
RB51	Vaccinated	36	1 a	2.7	0.4–14.1
	Control	36	0 a	0.0	0.0–0.09
RB51-SOD	Vaccinated	36	2 a	5.5	1.5–18.1
	Control	36	0 a	0.0	0.0–0.09

Different superscripts indicate statistical difference by column (P< 0.01).

Table 3.
Seroconvertion rates determined by RBPT at 30 days after vaccination of goats with Rev-1, RB51, and RB51-SOD strains in Xaltepec, Perote, Veracruz, Mexico.

a prevalence of 2.7% and 5.5% (95%CI: 0.4–14.1 and 1.5–18.1, respectively). At 365 days post vaccination, only 11.1% of vaccinated animals with RB51 remained reacting; there were no seroreactors to RB51-SOD strain by RBPT. Meanwhile, animals vaccinated with RB51 and RB51-SOD did not produce anti-O side-chain antibodies as measured by RBPT. Non-vaccinated control goats were seronegative. The seroconversion of a vaccine is the persistent serological reaction, especially when animals are vaccinated as adults; these persistent serological reactions are mainly against the antigenic O-chain of the lipopolysaccharide present in smooth *Brucella* strains [20].

Tables 7–10 show positive animals to RBPT that were confirmed with the SRD at 30, 60, 90, and 365 days after vaccination. Only 2.7% (95%CI: 0.4–14.1) of goats

Group/subgroup		N	Time after vaccination (days)		
			60		
			Positive	Seroconversion rate (%)	95%CI
Rev 1	Vaccinated	36	27 a	72.2	56.0–84.1
	Control	36	4 b	11.1	4.4–25.3
RB51	Vaccinated	36	1 a	2.7	0.4–14.1
	Control	36	0 a	0.0	0.0–0.09
RB51-SOD	Vaccinated	36	2 a	5.5	1.5–18.1
	Control	36	0 a	0.0	0.0–0.09

Different superscripts indicate statistical difference by column (P< 0.01).

Table 4.
Seroconvertion rates determined by RBPT at 60 days after vaccination of goats with Rev-1, RB51, and RB51-SOD strains in Xaltepec, Perote, Veracruz, Mexico.

Group/subgroup		N	Time after vaccination (days)		
			90		
			Positive	Seroconversion rate (%)	95%CI
Rev 1	Vaccinated	36	23 a	63.8	47.5–77.5
	Control	36	4 b	11.1	4.4–25.3
RB51	Vaccinated	36	1 a	2.7	0.4–14.1
	Control	36	0 a	0.0	0.0–0.09
RB51-SOD	Vaccinated	36	2 a	5.5	1.5–18.1
	Control	36	0 a	0.0	0.0–0.09

Different superscripts indicate statistical difference by column (P< 0.01).

Table 5.
Seroconvertion rates determined by RBPT at 90 days after vaccination of goats with Rev-1, RB51, and RB51-SOD strains in Xaltepec, Perote, Veracruz, Mexico.

Group/subgroup		N	Time after vaccination (days)		
			365		
			Positive	Seroconversion rate (%)	95%CI
Rev 1	Vaccinated	36	5 a	13.8	6.0–28.6
	Control	36	9 a	25.0	13.7–41.0
RB51	Vaccinated	36	4 a	11.1	4.4–25.3
	Control	36	9 a	25.0	13.7–41.0
RB51-SOD	Vaccinated	36	0 a	0.0	0.0–0.09
	Control	36	7 a	19.4	9.7–35.0

Different superscripts indicate statistical difference by column (P< 0.01).

Table 6.
Seroconvertion rates determined by RBPT at 365 days after vaccination of goats with Rev-1, RB51, and RB51-SOD strains in Xaltepec, Perote, Veracruz, Mexico.

vaccinated with Rev. 1 became positive during the first three samplings, but this situation did not persist until at 365 days post vaccination as expected. Also, goats vaccinated with RB51 and RB51-SOD during the first 90 days post vaccination expressed

Group/subgroup		Time after vaccination (days)		
		30		
		Positive	Prevalence rate (%)	95%CI
Rev 1	Vaccinated	1/28	2.7	0.49–14.1
	Control	0/4	0.0	0.0–0.49
RB51	Vaccinated	0/1	0.0	0.0–0.79
	Control	0/0	w.d.*	w.d.*
RB51-SOD	Vaccinated	0/2	0.0	0.0–0.66
	Control	0/0	w.d.*	w.d.*

**w.d. = without data*

Table 7.
Seroconversion rates determined by SRD at 30 days after vaccination of goats with Rev-1, RB51, and RB51-SOD strains in Xaltepec, Perote, Veracruz, Mexico.

Group/subgroup		Time after vaccination (days)		
		60		
		Positive	Prevalence rate (%)	95%CI
Rev 1	Vaccinated	1/27	2.7	0.49–14.1
	Control	0/4	0.0	0.0–0.49
RB51	Vaccinated	0/1	0.0	0.0–0.79
	Control	0/0	w.d.*	w.d.*
RB51-SOD	Vaccinated	0/2	0.0	0.0–0.66
	Control	0/0	w.d.*	w.d.*

**w.d. = without data*

Table 8.
Seroconversion rates determined by SRD at 60 days after vaccination of goats with Rev-1, RB51, and RB51-SOD strains in Xaltepec, Perote, Veracruz, Mexico.

Group/subgroup		Time after vaccination (days)		
		90		
		Positive	Prevalence rate (%)	95%CI
Rev 1	Vaccinated	1/23	2.7	0.49–14.1
	Control	0/4	0.0	0.0–0.49
RB51	Vaccinated	0/1	0.0	0.0–0.79
	Control	0/0	w.d.*	w.d.*
RB51-SOD	Vaccinated	0/2	0.0	0.0–0.66
	Control	0/0	w.d.*	w.d.*

**w.d. = without data*

Table 9.
Seroconversion rates determined by SRD at 90 days after vaccination of goats with Rev-1, RB51, and RB51-SOD strains in Xaltepec, Perote, Veracruz, Mexico.

antibodies that were detected with the RBPT test but were negative to the SRD test; however, at 365 days, an animal in the RB51 strain group was identified as seropositive (2.7%, 95%CI: 0.4–14.1). It is noteworthy that serological samples that underwent

Group/subgroup		Time after vaccination (days)		
		365		
		Positive	Prevalence rate (%)	95%CI
Rev 1	Vaccinated	0/5	0.0	0.0–0.43
	Control	0/9	0.0	0.0–0.29
RB51	Vaccinated	1/4	2.7	0.49–14.1
	Control	1/9	2.7	0.49–14.1
RB51-SOD	Vaccinated	0/0	w.d.*	w.d.*
	Control	1/7	2.7	0.49–14.1

**w.d. = without data*

Table 10.
Seroconversion rates determined by SRD at 365 days after vaccination of goats with Rev-1, RB51, and RB51-SOD strains in Xaltepec, Perote, Veracruz, Mexico.

the confirmatory test (SRD) correspond to animals that had a positive result to the screening test (RBPT); hence, the original sample size was not decreased.

4. Discussion

Goat herds in the present study had similar conditions of feeding, handling, and confinement. Each group was exposed to animals infected with *Brucella* spp. Overall seroprevalence in the herds under study was 21.4% (95%CI: 18.1–25.1) with 3% RBST as screening and 1.2% (95%CI: 0.5–2.7) by SRD as the confirmatory one. These seroprevalences are similar to those found by Román-Ramírez et al. in 14 municipalities in the central area of the state of Veracruz, Mexico, that were 18.18% (95%CI: 15.15–21.64) by RBST and 0.52% (95%CI: 0.13–1.65) by SDR tests [12]. However, the seroprevalence is also greater than 9.8% reported by Solorio-Rivera et al. (95%CI: 8.8–10.7) [5] using RBST test in goat herds of the state of Michoacán, Mexico. This shows that the herds located in the community of Xaltepec, municipality of Perote, Veracruz, Mexico, have animals that could be exposed to brucellosis and the conditions of management provide an opportunity for the perpetuating the infection.

The permanent vaccination program for goat herds has been operating in the area since 1994 achieving the requirements for the control phase according to the Official Mexican Standard (NOM-041-ZOO-1995) National Campaign against brucellosis in animals. These findings may suggest that the vaccine used is not protecting all animals, the vaccine is not properly managed or injected, or vaccination is not timely applied, resulting in the possibility of maintaining infection in the animals. Furthermore, the animal may not develop the infection, but the immune response capability is then detected by the diagnostic screening test without being a truly infected animal. As a result, the recognized agglutination serological tests (RSBT) leads to diagnostic confusion determining infected animals to remain in the herds. Hence, it is necessary to evaluate the vaccine strain to be used in the brucellosis control programs, since the results shown in **Table 1** demonstrate that more than 50% of the animals reacted to the screening test, but are not infected as shown by the SRD test (**Tables 7–9**), which possess a greater sensitivity. This situation determines the need to invest in confirmatory tests [25–29].

When vaccinated groups of goats were evaluated by the RSBT, animals vaccinated with Rev. 1 strain had a seroconversion rate of 77.7% (95%CI: 61.9–88.2),

72.2% (95%CI: 56.0–84.1), 63.8% (95%CI: 47.5–77.5), and 13.8% (95%CI: 6.0–28.6) at 30, 60, 90, and 365 days post vaccination, respectively (**Tables 3–6**). This agrees with Blasco et al. [7] who pointed out that vaccination with a full dose (1×10^9 CFU/mL) may cause diagnostic interference and inconvenience to rely on vaccination as the only alternative for brucellosis eradication programs in goat herds [7, 27]. RBST-positive animals were confirmed by the SRD test, and only one animal resulted positive, representing 2.7% (95%CI: 0.4–14.1) (**Tables 7–9**). This indicates that the vaccine did not protect or that the animal was infected prior to vaccination, despite being negative at initial screening. Vaccinated animals were not challenged at a controlled dose of *Brucella melitensis*, since the challenge was through a natural exposure to the infected animals, which were kept in confinement with the vaccinated animals, to allow exposed vaccinated animals to become infected as occurring in the normal management situation in the regional production systems in Mexico [14, 30].

As observed in **Tables 3–5**, animals vaccinated with the RB51 and RB51-SOD strains, 2.7% (95%CI: 0.4–14.1) and 5.5% (95%CI: 1.5–18.1), respectively, reacted to the RBST during the evaluation period. However, when analyzed by the SRD for confirmation, all animals were negative. RB51 strain is officially used for vaccination only in bovine females; it is a rough mutant strain derived from *B. abortus* 2308 smooth strain, so it does not induce response of anti-LPS antibodies. It has the advantage of allowing conventional serological tests to be used for brucellosis diagnosis in animals, and its use is considered safe in small ruminants [31]. Fosgate et al. carried out a study in water buffalo males and females which were vaccinated subcutaneously with RB51 at a concentration of $1.0–3.4 \times 10^{10}$ UFC/mL, to evaluate the serological performance by agglutination tests [31]. Animals were challenged in a herd with an initial *Brucella* spp. prevalence of 56%. Out of the vaccinated animals, 2/32 (6.2%) reacted in different samplings in at least one serological test (STAT, SPAT, and/or BPAT). Authors conclude that the proportion of vaccinated animals that became positive to brucellosis in this field trial was greater than the corresponding proportion in the control group emphasizing that vaccination does not stop the seroconversion effect on the herds challenged with a field strain. Furthermore, the RB51 vaccine did not prevent seroconversion of the animals. Therefore, infected animals were able to process the agent and maintain such a condition that it could react to the diagnostic test by IgM production by stimulation of the O-type side chains of the field strain, although the animal was not infected [28, 29, 32].

El Idrissi et al. compared the vaccine efficacy of Rev. 1 and RB51 strains in sheep. Considering seroconversion, they conclude that after vaccination, all sheep vaccinated with Rev. 1 were positive to RBPT and complement fixation test (CFT) at 2 weeks, reaching their maximum between 2 and 6 weeks [7]. Then the percentage decreased and was zero 14 weeks after challenge. Animals vaccinated with RB51 did not produce anti-O side-chain antibodies, as measured by RBPT and CFT. After exposure to challenge, anti-O side-chain antibodies, measured by RBPT, were detected in the serum of vaccinated animals and controls [19].

Out of the animals vaccinated with RB51-SOD strain, 2/36 were seroconverted, representing 5.5% (95%CI: 1.5–18.1) (**Tables 3–5**). The animals that underwent the confirmatory test (SRD) were negative as shown in **Tables 7–9**. The above indicates that animals established an immune memory response generating the production of immunoglobulins detectable by the screening test, but they were not infected [34]. Olsen et al. [32] evaluated the RB51-SOD strain in bisons, which was less effective than RB51 in protecting against abortion and uterine infection in this species [32–34]. In the present study, some animals of the goat groups of *B. abortus* strains RB51 and RB51-SOD were positive only to the screening test, which could be discarded by SRD test that identified them as negative to brucellosis [28, 29, 31, 33, 34].

The RB51-SOD strain was obtained from *B. abortus* 2308 in order to generate the overexpression of a protective periplasmic antigen of the protective antigen known as Cu/Zn SOD, which causes the immune cell response by T-helper-type Th1 lymphocytes, and protection against the strain of *B. abortus* 2308, which has been demonstrated in murine models [26, 29, 31–33]. Despite the favorable outcome in mice, Dorneles et al. [33] pointed out that the potential use of RB51-SOD under field conditions is very limited, although satisfactory results have been obtained. It is important to consider that the response observed in the mice might not reflect the protection achieved in the natural hosts after vaccination. Moreover, to generate a strong and protective immune response that mimic natural infection is a complex challenge. However, the current study in goats allowed to evaluate the RB51-SOD strain and to know part of its satisfactory performance in the field, since the newly developed vaccines have only evaluated in murine models [28–30]. Contrary to the Rev. 1 vaccine, current study demonstrates that the RB51-SOD strain does not induce seroconversion in goats.

5. Conclusion

When evaluating the Rev. 1, RB51, and RB51-SOD vaccine strains, seroconversion in animals vaccinated with Rev. 1 strain was higher than that shown by the strains RB51 and RB51-SOD by conventional serological tests in infected herds during the evaluated period. Therefore, vaccination with Rev. 1 originates the need to perform confirmatory tests causing an increase in diagnosis costs. According to results of the present study, the RB51-SOD vaccine represents an alternative for controlling one of the most important worldwide zoonosis in goats. However, further studies are required to evaluate the performance of immune response, vaccine safety, and efficacy at field level.

Acknowledgements

We thank the state committee for the promotion and protection of livestock of Veracruz and the product system goats of Veracruz. This work was supported by SEP-PRODEP research grant project [DSA/I103.5/I5/14220] “Support for the integration of thematic networks of academic collaboration.”

Conflict of interest

The authors have no conflict of interest to declare.

Author details

Baldomero Molina-Sánchez[1], David I. Martínez-Herrera[1]*, Violeta T. Pardío-Sedas[1], Ricardo Flores-Castro[2], José F. Morales-Álvarez[2] and José A. Villagómez-Cortés[1]

1 Facultad de Medicina Veterinaria y Zootecnia, Universidad Veracruzana, Veracruz, Veracruz, México

2 Centro Nacional de Investigación Disciplinaria Microbiología (CENID-Microbiología), Instituto Nacional de Investigaciones Forestales, Agrícolas y Pecuarias, Santa Fé, Ciudad de México, México

*Address all correspondence to: dmartinez@uv.mx

References

[1] Gul ST, Khan A. Epidemiology and epizootology of brucellosis: A review. Pakistan Veterinary Journal. 2007;**27**:145-151

[2] Arenas-Gamboa AM, Rossetti CA, Chaki SP, Garcia-Gonzalez DG, Adams LG, Ficht TA. Human brucellosis and adverse pregnancy outcomes. Current Tropical Medicine Reports. 2016;**3**:164-172

[3] Kaltungo BY, Saidu SNA, Musa IW, Baba AY. Brucellosis: A neglected zoonosis. British Microbiology Research Journal. 2014;**4**:1551-1574

[4] Reviriego FJ, Moreno MA, Domınguez L. Risk factors for brucellosis seroprevalence of sheep and goat flocks in Spain. Preventive Veterinary Medicine. 2000;**44**:167-173

[5] Solorio-Rivera JL, Segura-Correa JC, Sánchez-Gil LG. Seroprevalence of and risk factors for brucellosis of goats in herds of Michoacan, Mexico. Preventive Veterinary Medicine. 2007;**82**(3):282-290

[6] Lopez-Merino AH, Migrañas-Ortiz R, Perez-Miravete A, Magos C, Izaba BS, Tapia-Coyner R, et al. Seroepidemiología de la brucelosis en México. Salud Pública de México. 1992;**34**(2):230-240

[7] Blasco JM, Molina-Flores B. Control and eradication of *Brucella melitensis* infection in sheep and goats. Veterinary Clinics of North America: Food Animal Practice. 2011;**27**(1):95-104

[8] Montiel DO, Frankena K, Udo H, Baer NMK, Van der Zijpp A. Prevalence and risk factors for brucellosis in goats in areas of Mexico with and without brucellosis control campaign. Tropical Animal Health and Production. 2013;**45**(6):1383-1389

[9] Mendez-Lozano M, Rodríguez-Reyes EJ, Sánchez-Zamorano LM. Brucelosis, una zoonosis presente en la población: estudio de series de tiempo en México. Salud Pública México. 2015;**57**:519-527

[10] Tsegay A, Tuli G, Kassa T, Kebede N. Seroprevalence and risk factors of Brucellosis in small ruminants slaughtered at Debre Ziet and Modjo export abattoirs, Ethiopia. Journal of Infection in Developing Countries. 2015;**9**:373-380

[11] Wareth G, Melzer F, Elschner MC, Neubauer H, Roesler U. Detection of *Brucella melitensis* in bovine milk and milk products from apparently healthy animals in Egypt by real-time PCR. Journal of Infection in Developing Countries. 2014;**8**(10):1339-1343

[12] Román-Ramírez DL, Martínez-Herrera DI, Villagómez-Cortés JAJ, Peniche-Cardeña ÁE, Morales-Álvarez JF, Flores-Castro R. Epidemiología de la brucelosis caprina en la Zona Centro del Estado de Veracruz. Gaceta Médica de México. 2017;**153**(1):26-30

[13] Villa R, Perea M, Aparicio ED, Mobarak AS, Andrade LH, Güemes FS. Abortions and stillbirths in goats immunized against brucellosis using RB51, rfbK and Rev 1 vaccines. Tecnica Pecuaria en Mexico. 2008;**46**(3):249-257

[14] Schurig GG, Sriranganathan N, Corbel MJ. Brucellosis vaccines: past, present and future. Veterinary Microbiology. 2002;**90**(1):479-496

[15] Luna-Martínez JE, Mejía-Terán C. Brucellosis in Mexico: Current status and trends. Veterinary Microbiology. 2002;**90**(1):19-30

[16] El Idrissi AH, Benkirane A, El Maadoudi M, Bouslikhane M, Berrada J, Zerouali A. Comparison of the efficacy

of *Brucella abortus* strain RB51 and *Brucella melitensis* Rev. 1 live vaccines against experimental infection with *Brucella melitensis* in pregnant ewes. Revue Scientifique et Technique-Office International des Épizooties. 2001;**20**(3):741-744

[17] Poester FP, Ramos ET, Gomes MJP, Chiminazzo C, Schurig G. The serological response of adult cattle after vaccination with *Brucella abortus* strain 19 and RB51. Brazilian Journal of Veterinary Research and Animal Science. 2000;**37**(1)

[18] Garin-Bastuji B, Blasco JM, Marín C, Albert D. The diagnosis of brucellosis in sheep and goats, old and new tools. Small Ruminant Research. 2006;**62**(1):63-70

[19] Rahman S, Baek BK. Diagnostic efficacy of *Brucella abortus* strain RB51 in experimentally inoculated Sprague-Dawley rats using western blot assay. Journal of Infection in Developing Countries. 2008;**2**(05):384-388

[20] Mikolon AB, Gardner IA, Hietala SK, de Anda JH, Pestaña EC, Hennager SG, et al. Evaluation of North American antibody detection tests for diagnosis of brucellosis in goats. Journal of Clinical Microbiology. 1998;**36**(6):1716-1722

[21] Garin – Bastuji B, Blasco JM, Marín C, Albert D. The diagnosis of brucellosis in sheep and goats, old and new tolos. Small Ruminant Research. 2006;**62**:63-70

[22] Coelho AM, Díez JG, Coelho AC. Brucelosis en pequeños rumiantes: efecto de la aplicación de un programa especial de vacunación en masa con REV-1. Revista electrónica de Veterinaria. 2013;**14**(12):1-16

[23] Thrusfield M. Veterinary Epidemiology. 3rd ed. UK: Blackwell Science Oxford; 2005

[24] Campbell MJ, Machin D, Walters SJ. Medical Statistics: A Textbook for the Health Sciences. 4th ed. Chichester, West Sussex, England: John Wiley & Sons; 2010. pp. 89-93

[25] Ali S, Akhter S, Neubauer H, Melzer F, Khan I, Ali Q, et al. Serological, cultural, and molecular evidence of Brucella infection in small ruminants in Pakistan. Journal of Infection in Developing Countries. 2015;**9**(05):470-475

[26] Blasco JM. Existing and future vaccines against brucellosis in small ruminants. Small Ruminant Research. 2006;**62**(1):33-37

[27] Martínez Martínez OL, Pérez De la Rosa R, Díaz Aparicio E, Snyderlaar Hardwicke AC, Hernández Andrade L, Suárez Güemes F. Estudio de la eliminación en la leche de la cepa Rev 1 de *Brucella melitensis* en cabras vacunadas con dosis reducida. Tecnica Pecuaria en Mexico. 2005;**43**(3):399-404

[28] Yang X, Skyberg JA, Cao L, Clapp B, Thornburg T, Pascual DW. Progress in Brucella vaccine development. Frontiers of Biology. 2013;**8**(1):60-77

[29] Fosgate GT, Adesiyun AA, Hird DW, Johnson WO, Hietala SK, Schurig GG, et al. Evaluation of brucellosis RB51 vaccine for domestic water buffalo (*Bubalus bubalis*) in Trinidad. Preventive Veterinary Medicine. 2003;**58**(3):211-225

[30] Vemulapalli R, He Y, Cravero S, Sriranganathan N, Boyle SM, Schurig GG. Overexpression of protective antigen as a novel approach to enhance vaccine efficacy of *Brucella abortus* strain RB51. Infection and Immunity. 2000;**68**(6):3286-3289

[31] Oñate AA, Céspedes S, Cabrera A, Rivers R, González A, Muñoz C,

et al. A DNA vaccine encoding Cu, Zn superoxide dismutase of *Brucella abortus* induces protective immunity in BALB/c mice. Infection and Immunity. 2003;**71**(9):4857-4861

[32] Olsen SC, Boyle SM, Schurig GG, Sriranganathan NN. Immune responses and protection against experimental challenge after vaccination of bison with *Brucella abortus* strain RB51 or RB51 overexpressing superoxide dismutase and glycosyltransferase genes. Clinical and Vaccine Immunology. 2009;**16**(4):535-540

[33] Dorneles EM, Sriranganathan N, Lage AP. Recent advances in *Brucella abortus* vaccines. Veterinary Research. 2015;**46**(1):76

[34] Goodwin ZI, Pascual DW. Brucellosis vaccines for livestock. Veterinary Immunology and Immunopathology. 2016;**181**:51-58

Chapter 3

Kidney Disease in Brucellosis

Shokoufeh Savaj

Abstract

Brucellosis, a prevalent zoonosis disease in different countries, can involve the kidney during infection and also present in the complicated form in hemodialysis (HD), peritoneal dialysis (PD), and kidney transplant (Tx) patient. In spite of few reports of kidney involvements in the literature, this infection can imitate a wide range of glomerular disease from minimal change, membranous glomeropathy, focal and diffuse proliferative glomerular disease to rapidly progressive glomerulonephritis. Cryoglobulinemia, thrombotic microangiopathy, and ANCA-associated glomerular disease are vasculitis form of the disease. Tubulointerstitial involvement, electrolyte disorder, renal abscess, and pyelonephritis can present the same as other Gram-negative infections. Moreover, peritonitis in PD patient, spondyloarthropathy in HD, and severe infection in kidney Tx patients have been reported. Infection recurrence and infection from kidney donors are another dilemma in renal recipients. Brucellosis as a multifaced disease can mimic a wide range of presentations in nephrology. Clinicians should keep in mind the diverse pictures of the disease, especially when they practice in the endemic area.

Keywords: kidney, brucellosis, glomerular disease, dialysis, kidney transplant

1. Introduction

Brucellosis, a prevalent zoonosis disease with a worldwide distribution, can involve the kidney during infection. In 1889, Bruce [1] firstly reported kidney disease in Malt fever. Since then, a wide range of kidney involvements from direct invasion of Brucella with abscess and tubulointerstitial nephritis, immune complex disease, vasculitis, and drug toxicity have been reported. Brucella infection in immunocompromised patient can induce a confusing picture with peritonitis in peritoneal dialysis (PD), spondylodiscitis in hemodialysis, and complicated form of the disease in kidney transplant (TX) patients. Immunosuppressive monitoring, drug side effects, and donor to recipient transmission or recurrence are great challenges in the management of organ recipients with brucellosis. In this chapter, different presentations of brucellosis in kidney including glomeruli, tubulointerstitial, and vasculature involvement are discussed. Secondly, the Brucella infection in PD, HD, and Tx patients are reviewed, and finally, the chance of infection transmission of Brucellosis in the donor and recipients and the challenging point of pretransplant evaluation in donors and recipients are discussed.

2. Glomerular disease in brucellosis

Glomerular disease is an uncommon presentation in brucellosis. It can present with hematuria, pyuria, proteinuria, increased blood pressure, edema, and renal failure. Glomerular involvement from mild proteinuria, microscopic hematuria up to the severe presentations of glomerular disease including rapidly progressive glomerulitis resulted in end-stage kidney disease have been reported. Glomeruli affected by immune complexes or vasculitis during Brucella endocarditis. The usual glomerulopathy in cases with endocarditis is focal and diffuse proliferative glomerulonephritis which are presented in the literature as membranoproliferative [2] and rapidly progressive glomerulonephritis; IgA nephropathy reported in two patients [3, 4] with proteinuria and hematuria. Siegelmann et al. [4] reported a case with nephrotic range proteinuria (6.0–13.0 g/day) and focal and segmental glomerulonephritis with mesangial proliferation and heavy deposit of IgA. Proteinuria persisted 3 months after completion of therapy, which indicates a secondary form of IgA nephropathy. Minimal change disease is a rare presentation of brucellosis reported only in one case without endocarditis. The patient had massive proteinuria who received prednisolone and antimicrobial treatment with complete remission and no recurrence after 1 year [5]. Membranous nephropathy is also diagnosed in one case with proteinuria [6].

3. Vasculitis in brucellosis

Vasculitis is a lethal picture of brucellosis with systemic organ involvement. Turgay et al. [7] reported 52-year-old male with Brucella infection and ANCA-associated vasculitis that induced rapidly progressive glomerulitis. The patient had endocarditis with vegetation on the aortic valve and leukocytoclastic vasculitis. Serology showed a high titer of serum agglutinin for Brucella and positive P-ANCA test. The patient recovered with combination therapy of plasmapheresis, methylprednisolone pulse, and antibiotic therapy. The other vasculitis form of kidney disease is cryoglobulinemia. This systemic disease can happen in malignancy, autoimmune, and infectious disease. Mixed cryoglobulinemia in brucellosis has been reported in five cases (four from Peru and one from Spain). They had a high polyclonal cryoglobulin level (IgG, IgA, and IgM) with a female preponderance (4:1). Four cases had positive bone marrow culture and one diagnosed based on serology [8]. Thrombotic microangiopathy that presents with microangiopathic hemolytic anemia, thrombocytopenia, and variable signs of organ impairment due to platelet aggregation in the microcirculation has been reported in patients with brucellosis. Erdem et al. [9] reported a 51-year-old man with thrombotic microangiopathy, hematuria, diminished consciousness, and renal failure. The patient received combination therapy with antimicrobials and plasma exchange with a good response and no recurrence in 1.5 years follow-up.

4. Tubulointerstitial and parenchymal involvement in brucellosis

Direct invasion of parenchyma and abscess formation is a rare manifestation of Brucella, which has been reported in five cases in the literature. Li et al. [10] reported a 45-year-old man with fever and flank pain. CT scan showed a low-density lesion in the right kidney in CT scan and positive culture for Brucella. He received 8 weeks course of treatment and relapse after discontinuation of treatment, which needed another 16 weeks course of rifampin and moxifloxacin for the eradication of bacteria. There are reports of acute interstitial nephritis [11] and pyelonephritis [12] after Brucella infection. A perplexing point is antimicrobial therapy with rifampin, which can induce interstitial nephritis. Salih et al. reported a 52-year-old man with a diagnosis of Brucella. Patient referred with acute renal failure 2 weeks after treatment with rifampin. Renal failure recovered since the drug was discontinued [13].

5. Electrolyte abnormality in Brucella infection

Syndrome of inappropriate secretion of ADH (SIADH), which presented with hyponatremia in a euvolemic patient without other electrolyte abnormality has been reported in patients with brucellosis. Bala et al. [14] in a study of 160 children and adolescent with SIADH reported 21.9% prevalence of SIADH. Urinary sodium (>25 mmol/L) with normal dietary salt intake, low uric acid (<2 mg/dL), the absence of kidney, thyroid or adrenal disease, and history of diuretic use were the criteria for diagnosis. Hyponatremia had a correlation to the severity of disease and managed with fluid restriction. Renal tubular disorder presented in 31 patients with active brucellosis [15]. They had phosphorus, potassium, and sodium handling abnormality in 31 patients. These patients were not malnourished, received fluid therapy, or hospitalized. They proposed that besides glomerular damage, tubular dysfunction is another presentation of Brucella infection.

6. Brucellosis in hemodialysis patients

Musculoskeletal problem is a prevalent feature in hemodialysis (HD) patients, which presents due to renal osteodystrophy and amyloidosis resulted from beta 2 microglobulin deposition in the joints. These symptoms can mislead the clinician to overlook Brucella diagnosis. Inversely, fever as a common presentation of the infectious disease is missing in those ill patients. Most of the reported cases of brucellosis in HD patients presented with musculoskeletal pain, arthralgia, low back pain, and malaise in the acute form of brucellosis. Paravertebral and epidural abscess with spondylodiscitis in thoracic and lumbar vertebra and neurobrucellosis with a headache, diplopia, and cranial nerve involvement were reported as the complicated chronic form brucellosis in HD patients [16]. There is also a report of fatal septicemia and endocarditis [17, 18] in HD patients. Blood cultures should be performed in HD patients when typical symptoms of brucellosis exist even when the patient has no fever. Drug toxicity and dose adjustment are the other obstacles in the treatment of these patients. Rifampin and doxycycline with a hepatic metabolism do not need any dose adjustment; however, aminoglycosides, cephalosporins, and fluoroquinolones should be prescribed based on patient's eGFR and patient needs a supplement dose after dialysis course.

7. Brucellosis in peritoneal dialysis (PD) patients

Peritoneal dialysis patients are at risk of peritonitis. Gram-positive organisms are the common cause of infections in 80% of the episodes. There are few reports of peritonitis due to Brucella infection in the literature. All of the cases presented with a typical peritoneal infection with neutrophil predominance with a positive culture in 5–21 days [19]. Organ involvement is hematogenous in most of the studies; however, Osizik et al. [20] showed a positive peritoneal fluid culture with a negative blood culture and serology. They proposed a direct inoculation of bacteria from the catheter to peritoneum based on the patient's occupation. The other issue in Brucella peritonitis in PD patients is any need for catheter removal after Brucella infection. Taskapan et al. [21] and Alothman et al. [22] reported two cases with a recurrence of infection in 6–8 weeks after treatment that resulted in catheter removal for complete eradication of bacteria. On the other hand, Unal et al. [23] and Solak et al. [19] in two different reports showed the complete cure of infection despite keeping peritoneal catheter. Drug regimen in these studies was 6 weeks course of rifampin and doxycycline.

8. Brucellosis in renal transplant recipients

However, the prevalence of brucellosis is around 1 in 500,000 population, and there are few reports in renal transplant recipients. In another view, these patients are at risk of different opportunistic infections. Most of the time, diagnosis of brucellosis was lately with the complicated form of the disease. There were two reports of neurobrucellosis in renal Tx patients in the literature, one with loss of consciousness and encephalitis [24] and the other one with a seizure and headache [25]. Endocarditis [26], pulmonary involvement [27], hepatobiliary and hematologic [28], pyelonephritis and dysuria [29], and arthritis [30] were other presentations of the disease. They were diagnosed based on serology or fluid culture that finally guided to the diagnosis of brucellosis. In addition to the complicated form of the disease and late diagnosis, drug interferences, especially calcineurin inhibitors, are another challenging point in the treatment of disease. Rifampin decreases drug level and inversely clarithromycin increases drug level that induces calcineurin toxicity. Hence, streptomycin with nephrotoxic nature cannot be the first choice in renal Tx patient. Ting et al. suggested tigecycline as an alternative drug in renal Tx patient. Triple antibacterial treatment has experienced in these immunocompromised patients with a complicated form of the disease [26, 30]. In these six reports, all of the patients completed the 6–12 weeks course of treatment with a good outcome and no recurrence; however, they experienced a serum creatinine rise.

9. Kidney donor evaluation before transplant

Evaluation for Brucella infection is suggested before organ transplantation in donors and recipients, especially in endemic areas. There are some reports of Brucella transmission and recurrence after liver [31], bone marrow transplantation [32, 33]. Serologic tests including serum agglutination and ELISA should be performed before organ transplant. Positive titers consisted of 1:80 in the non-endemic area and 1:160 in the endemic area are suspicious and needs further evaluation. Serologic tests are not enough to distinguish active and past infection, which needs more evaluation by infectious disease specialist.

10. Conclusion

In this chapter, a wide range of Brucella presentations was discussed. Brucellosis as a multifaced disease can imitate a large group of non-infectious causes of kidney disease. Hence, the misdiagnosis could be hazardous and end to the patient's morbidity and mortality. Clinicians should keep in mind the diverse pictures of the disease, especially when they practice in the endemic area.

Author details

Shokoufeh Savaj
Internal Medicine Department, Branch of Nephrology, Iran University of Medical Sciences, Firoozgar Hospital, Tehran, Iran

*Address all correspondence to: savaj.sh@iums.ac.ir

References

[1] Bruce DJ. Observations on Malta fever. BMJ. 1101;**1**(1481):1889

[2] Provatopoulou S, Papasotiriou M, Papachristou E, Gakiopoulou H, Marangos M, Goumenos DS, et al. Membranoproliferative glomerulonephritis in a patient with chronic brucellosis. Kidney Research and Clinical Practice. 2018;**37**(3):298

[3] Ardalan MR, Shoja MM. Rapidly progressive glomerulonephritis in a patient with brucellosis. Nephrology Dialysis Transplantation. 2006;**21**(6):1743-1744

[4] Siegelmann N, Abraham A, Rudensky B, Shemesh OJ. Brucellosis with nephrotic syndrome, nephritis, and IgA nephropathy. Postgraduate Medical Journal. 1992;**68**(804):834-836

[5] Sabanis N, Gavriilaki E, Paschou E, Tsotsiou E, Kalaitzoglou A, Kavlakoudis C, et al. Renal manifestations of human brucellosis: First report of minimal change disease. Saudi Journal of Kidney Disease and Transplantation. 2016;**27**(3):590

[6] Eugene M, Gauvain J, Roux C, Barthez J. A case of acute brucellosis with membranous glomerulopathy. Clinical Nephrology. 1987;**28**(3):158

[7] Turgay M, Ertuğrul E, Küçükşahin O, Şahin A. Brucellosis with p-ANCA-associated renal failure, leukocytoclastic vasculitis and endocarditis: Case report. Journal of Microbiology and Infectious Diseases. 2011;**1**(01):31-34

[8] Delgado S, Bravo F, Gotuzzo E. Mixed cryoglobulinemia due to brucellosis. Clinical Infectious Diseases. 2008;**47**(3):435-436

[9] Erdem F, Kiki İ, Gündoğdu M, Kaya H. Thrombotic thrombocytopenic purpura in a patient with Brucella infection is highly responsive to combined plasma infusion and antimicrobial therapy. Medical Principles and Practice. 2007;**16**(4):324-326

[10] Li J, Li Y, Wang Y, Huo N, Wan H, Lin X, et al. Renal abscess caused by Brucella. International Journal of Infectious Diseases. 2014;**28**:26-28

[11] Patino R, Blanco J, Yubero B. Interstitial nephritis caused by Brucella. Revista Clínica Española. 1973;**129**(1):93-96

[12] Honey RM, Gelfand M, Myers NH. Chronic brucella pyelonephritis with calcification: Short review of the literature and report of a case. Central African Journal of Medicine. 1957

[13] Salih SB, Kharal M, Qahtani M, Dahneem L, Nohair S. Acute interstitial nephritis induced by intermittent use of rifampicin in patient with brucellosis. Saudi Journal of Kidney Diseases and Transplantation. 2008;**19**(3):450-452

[14] Bala KA, Doğan M, Kaba S, Akbayram S, Aslan O, Kocaman S, et al. The syndrome of inappropriate secretion of anti-diuretic hormone (SIADH) and brucellosis. Medical Science Monitor. 2016;**22**:3129

[15] Conkar S, Kosker M, Cevik S, Ay M. Association of brucellosis with renal tubular and glomerular damage in children in Turkey. Saudi Journal of Kidney Diseases and Transplantation. 2018;**29**(2):284

[16] Turunç T, Demiroğlu YZ, Alişkan H, Çolakoğlu Ş, Timurkaynak F, Özdemir N, et al. Brucellosis in cases of end-stage renal disease. Nephrology Dialysis Transplantation. 2008;**23**(7):2344-2349

[17] Sungur C, Sungur A, Gedikoglu G, Usubutun A, Yasavul U, Turgan C, et al. Fatal *Brucella melitensis* endocarditis

in a hemodialysis patient. Nephron. 1994;**67**(2):234-235

[18] Stich-Kreitner V, Piper C, Schassan H. A rare cause of infection in chronic dialysis patients: Malta fever (febris undulans melitensis). Klinische Wochenschrift. 1988;**66**(16):743-746

[19] Solak Y, Biyik Z, Demircioglu S, Polat I, Genc N, Turkmen K, et al. *Brucella peritonitis* in peritoneal dialysis: A case report and review of the literature. Peritoneal Dialysis International. 2012;**32**(2):126-130

[20] Ozisik L, Akman B, Huddam B, Azap OK, Bilgic A, Sezer S, et al. Isolated *Brucella peritonitis* in a CAPD patient. American Journal of Kidney Diseases. 2006;**47**(5):e65-ee6. DOI: 10.1136/bcr-2018-225865

[21] Taskapan H, Oymak O, Sümerkan B, Tokgoz B, Utas C. *Brucella peritonitis* in a patient on continuous ambulatory peritoneal dialysis with acute brucellosis. Nephron. 2002;**91**(1):156-158

[22] Alothman A, Al Khurmi A, Al Sadoon S, Alhejaili F. *Brucella peritonitis* in a patient on peritoneal dialysis. Saudi Journal of Kidney Diseases and Transplantation. 2008;**19**(3):428

[23] Taskapan H, Oymak O, Sümerkan B, Tokgoz B, Utas C. *Brucella peritonitis* in a patient on continuous ambulatory peritoneal dialysis with acute brucellosis. Nephron. May 2002;**91**(1):156-158

[24] Yousif B, Nelson J. Neurobrucellosis—A rare complication of renal transplantation. American Journal of Nephrology. 2001;**21**(1):66-68

[25] Alqwaifly M, Al-Ajlan FS, Al-Hindi H, Al Semari A. Central nervous system brucellosis granuloma and white matter disease in immunocompromised patient. Emerging Infectious Diseases. 2017;**23**(6):978

[26] Bishara J, Robenshtok E, Weinberger M, Yeshurun M, Sagie A, Pitlik S. Infective endocarditis in renal transplant recipients. Transplant Infectious Disease. 1999;**1**(2):138-143

[27] Ay N, Kaya S, Anil M, Alp V, Beyazit U, Yuksel E, Danis R. Pulmonary Involvement in Brucellosis, a Rare Complication of Renal Transplant: Case Report and Brief Review. 2016

[28] Ting IW, Ho MW, Sung YJ, Tien N, Chi CY, Ho HC, et al. Brucellosis in a renal transplant recipient. 2013;**15**(5):E191-E1E5

[29] Inayat F, Mahboob M, Ali NS, Bokhari SRA, Ashraf A. Brucellosis in renal transplant recipients: A comparative review of 5 cases. BMJ Case Reports. 2018;**2018**. DOI: 10.1136/bcr-2018-225865

[30] Einollahi B, Hajarizadeh B, Bakhtiari S, Lesanpezeshki M, Khatami MR, Nourbala MH, et al. Pretransplant hepatitis C virus infection and its effect on the post-transplant course of living renal allograft recipients. Journal of Gastroenterology and Hepatology. 2003;**18**(7):836-840

[31] Islek A, Sayar E, Yilmaz A, Günseren F, Artan R. Relapsing brucellosis after liver transplantation in a child: What is the appropriate regimen and duration of therapy? Transplantation. 2013;**96**(2):e6-e7

[32] Ertem M, Kürekçi A, Aysev D, Ünal E, Ikincioğulları A. Brucellosis transmitted by bone marrow transplantation. Bone Marrow Transplantation. 2000;**26**(2):225

[33] Tuon FF, Gondolfo RB, Cerchiari N. Human-to-human transmission of Brucella—A systematic review. Tropical Medicine & International Health. 2017;**22**(5):539-546

Chapter 4

Neonatal Brucellosis

Fatemeh Eghbalian

Abstract

Brucellosis is a zoonotic infectious disease caused by the *Brucella* bacteria. Neonatal brucellosis is very rare and preventable and is an example of intrauterine infection, but clinical manifestations as well as transmission route are not well defined but presumed transplacental transmission. The neonate can be either infected transplacentally, or by ingestion of mother's secretions and blood during delivery, or by ingestion of breast milk. Presentation of the neonatal brucellosis including fever, arthralgia, weakness, malaise, respiratory distress, pneumonia, enlargement of liver and spleen, fever, thrombocytopenia, late neonatal hyperbilirubinemia, and septicoemia. The diagnosis of brucellosis was based on a positive blood culture (isolation *Brucella* of blood culture from both the mother and the neonate or only neonate) and on a high or rising titer of antibodies to the *Brucella* organism (positive serology only in the mother or both). The neonates with negative *Brucella* serology may also have *Brucella* infection. The mortality rate is very high, and infected neonates need early detection and timely treatment. Early detection and treatment reduce the incidence of complications. The treatment of rifampicin and trimethoprim/sulfamethoxazole is useful for neonatal brucellosis. More patients with neonatal brucellosis well respond to antibiotic therapy and must monitor by a *Brucella* titer of <1:40.

Keywords: neonate, brucellosis, congenital

1. Introduction

Brucellosis is one of the most widespread zoonoses world [1, 2]. It is an acute or chronic zoonotic infection usually transmitted to humans through direct contact with infected animals or by eating contaminated food from infected animals (cattle, sheep, goats, pigs, or another animals) or food products such as unpasteurized milk, cheese or inhalation of contaminated air or dust particles and exposure is frequently occupational [1–4]. The prevalence of brucellosis has been increasing due to growing international tourism and migration of peoples [5, 6]. It is an important cause of economic loss and public health problems and is one of the important human infections in many developing countries or parts of the world. Brucellosis affects humans in all age groups and both genders with variable incidence according to the geographic location and the strain [1–43]. Although this disease is now uncommon in the United States and Britain but common in the Latin America, Africa, Mediterranean and Persian Gulf regions and parts of Asia specially in Iran [1–8, 32, 39]. Brucellosis has high morbidity both for animals or humans and one of the causes of abortion in animals but in humans it causes multisystem disease [1–8, 44]. Brucellosis is not uncommon in many parts of the world but human-to-human transmission, for example, through sexual intercourse, mother to newborn is rare, but possible and has been reported [9–11]. Vertical transmission from mother to fetus during pregnancy (transplacental) or perinatal exposure has been reported [7, 8, 12, 13, 16–18, 25, 44]. Other modes of human-to-human transmission of brucellosis include blood transfusion, bone marrow transplantation and breastfeeding [20–25]. Although few cases of perinatal brucellosis have been reported but the mode of transmission of *Brucella* from the mother to the baby remains uncertain.

2. Neonatal brucellosis

Brucellosis is a primarily zoonotic infection, public health problem and serious threat for people living in endemic areas of world which is caused by Gram-negative, intracellular, non-spore-forming, non-capsulated, aerobic, nonmotile *Coccobacilli* [1, 26–41]. *Brucella melitensis* is the most important species for human brucellosis, but other species, including *B. abortus*, *B. suis*, *B. canis*, and *B. novel* marine have also been associated with human cases [1–3, 26, 29, 32 43]. Brucellosis can be transmitted to humans from direct contact by infected animals, products of conception, or animal discharge, and by consumption of infected milk, milk products or meat [2, 3, 5, 26, 32, 43]. Human-to-human transmission is rare, but has been reported in association with blood transfusions, bone marrow transplantation, trans placental or perinatal exposure and possibly postnatally by consumption breast feeding [7, 8, 12, 13, 16–18, 20–25, 44].

Neonatal brucellosis is rare and there are only a few reports of congenital brucellosis [7, 8, 12–14, 17, 43, 44]. There are few data supporting transmission from mother to fetus or transmission via breast milk [7, 8, 12, 13, 16–18, 23, 25]. It seems that in most cases *Brucella* passes through the placenta. Transplacental and consumption breast milk are the main routes of *Brucella* transmission in mammalian reservoirs [7, 8, 12, 13, 23–25]. Ingestion of maternal blood, urine or feces during delivery might be another rout of *Brucella* transmission [10, 14, 19].

Although infected pregnant animals transfer *Brucella* to their offspring transplacentally with resultant massive wastage of conception, this mode of transmission and resultant interference with the normal course of pregnancy has been disputed in humans [2, 32, 43].

Neonatal brucellosis is a very rare cause of early onset neonatal sepsis but should be considered in neonates born from mothers at risk for brucellosis [7–10]. Physicians dealing with mothers who lived in endemic areas during pregnancy should maintain a large index of suspicion when these mothers present with unexplained symptoms, especially for those with social and occupational risk for brucellosis because as soon as diagnosis and therapy can lead to good and better outcome. Education for pregnant women living in endemic areas for avoidance of exposure to sheep, goat, camels and do not consumption of unpasteurized products is most important and highly recommended. Family history of brucellosis or exposure must be obtained during prenatal care in endemic areas [1, 38, 39]. Sometimes maternal brucellosis lead to preterm delivery and with adverse long-term outcomes [16]. Transplacental transmissions from an infected mother, exposure to maternal blood, urine, or genital secretions during delivery are the main routes of transmission of neonatal brucellosis [10, 14, 19].

Pregnancy caused to impaired immunological status, and infection with *Brucella* can deformation obstetric outcomes, including congenital infection [44, 45]. At one point it was believed that adverse pregnancy outcomes associated with human brucellosis should be uncommon due to the absence of erythritol in the human placenta [46, 47]. Another theory was that amniotic fluid contains anti-*Brucella* activity [48]. However, many reports describe apparent increased rates of spontaneous abortion, intrauterine fetal death, and preterm birth in mothers with brucellosis during pregnancy [49]. Recognition and suitable treatment of infection in early course of pregnancy lead to decrease of incidence of spontaneous abortion, intrauterine fetal death, and congenital infection [44, 46–49]. The clinical manifestations of brucellosis in pregnancy are similar to other infected people and include arthralgia, arthritis, fever, chills, sweating, headache, malaise, nausea, vomiting, lymphadenopathy, hepatosplenomegaly, anorexia and weight loss [1–3, 45–47]. Positive blood or bone marrow culture are definite diagnosis but serologic tests (Wright and 2-mercapto ethanol, 2ME) are the commonest diagnostic methods [1, 3, 45–47].

The choice treatment for brucellosis in infected mother during pregnancy is a combination of rifampin and trimethoprim-sulfamethoxazole but trimethoprim-sulfamethoxazole is contraindicated in first trimester and the last 2–4 weeks of pregnancy. During the third generation and first trimester of pregnancy, cephalosporins have been used and in the last month of pregnancy, combination of aminoglycosides (gentamycin) with rifampin is an alternative regimen [33, 39, 45–49].

3. Clinical manifestations

Newborns with symptom onset in the first week of life have presumably congenital brucellosis, although the incubation period of *Brucella* in newborn period can vary from less 1 week to 1 months (typically 2–4 weeks) [50]. Delayed diagnosis of congenital brucellosis in preterm infants can overlap with other diseases of prematurity. Term infants with onset of symptoms beyond 1 week of age may have acquired *Brucella* through breastfeeding or ingestion of nonhuman milk but congenital infection can also have a delayed presentation [9]. The neonatal immune system is immature, the response to well-characterized infective processes varies from that described in older children and hence clinical manifestations may differ. Differential diagnosis between other bacterial infections in the newborn and brucellosis is difficult and presentations of brucellosis in the neonate are nonspecific and it is very difficult to distinguish brucellosis clinically from other bacterial infections. Fever, arthralgia, night sweating, anemia, bone marrow failure, jaundice, respiratory distress, vomiting, irritability, seizure, hepatosplenomegaly, dearie, skin rash, nausea, vomiting, malaise, poor feeding, failure to thrive (FTT) and distended abdomen are probable signs and symptoms in neonatal brucellosis [48]. The role of *Brucella* in myocarditis and hydrocephalus is difficult to determine both reported from neonates who acquired *Brucella* from breast milk [51, 52]. In summary, brucellosis should be considered as a possible cause of early or late onset sepsis in newborns presenting with fever, respiratory distress and hepatosplenomegaly in endemic regions [53].

4. Diagnosis

Hematological and biochemical tests used in neonatal sepsis are of limited value for the diagnosis of brucellosis [17, 18]. In brucellosis, the white blood cell count is often normal or low. In neonates suspect to brucellosis, the diagnosis was made by the unexpected isolation of *Brucella* from blood culture obtained from a sick neonate with suspected sepsis. Serologic tests are also important methods for clinical diagnosis but should be interpreted judiciously because of transplacental passage of maternal IgG antibodies [54]. A negative serologic test should never exclude the diagnosis, particularly in preterm neonates who may not have mounted their own antibody response nor received transplacental antibodies. For further evaluation, blood should be sent for nested PCR and DNA sequencing. Definite diagnosis in neonates could be verified based on separating etiologic agent since maternal IgG exists in infant serum till 6 months after delivery [7–9, 17, 18, 54].

5. Treatment

Tetracycline or doxycycline with streptomycin or gentamicin are recommended therapies in older children or adults [39, 55]. Quinolones and doxycycline are sometimes used for treatment of brucellosis in adolescents but their safety in infants and newborns has not been established [32, 33]. Because of the side effects of tetracycline and doxycycline in children younger than 10 years of age, a variety of drugs can be used safely, for example a combination of rifampin and trimethoprim-sulfamethoxazole [32, 33, 43, 55].

The combination of intravenous aminoglycosides for 5–7 days plus with rifampicin and trimethoprim-sulfamethoxazole orally 6–8 weeks is a commonly regimen and has been suggested as the treatment of choice for neonatal brucellosis [7, 8, 12, 13, 56].

Author details

Fatemeh Eghbalian
Department of Pediatrics, Hamadan University of Medical Sciences, Hamedan, Iran

*Address all correspondence to: eghbalian_fa@yahoo.com

References

[1] Bosilkovski M, Dimzova M, Grozdanovski K. Natural history of brucellosis in an endemic region in different time periods. Acta Clinica Croatica. 2009;**48**:41

[2] Young EJ. *Brucella* species. In: Mandelle G, Bennet J, Dolin R, editors. Principles and Practices of Infections Diseases, 6th edition, Strickland GT (Ed), Churchill Livingstone, Philadelphia; 2005. pp. 2669-2674

[3] Wright SG. Brucellosis. In: Strickland GT, editor. Hunter's Tropical Medicine and Emerging Infectious Diseases. 8th ed. Philadelphia: W.B. Saunders Company; 2000. p. 416

[4] Mesner O, Riesenberg K, Biliar N, et al. The many faces of human-to-human transmission of brucellosis: Congenital infection and outbreak of nosocomial disease related to an unrecognized clinical case. Clinical Infectious Diseases. 2007;**45**:e135-e140

[5] Godfroid J, Cloeckaert A, Liautard JP, et al. From the discovery of the Malta fever's agent to the discovery of a marine mammal reservoir, brucellosis has continuously been a re-emerging zoonosis. Veterinary Research. 2005;**36**:313

[6] Bricker BJ, Ewalt DR, MacMillan AP, et al. Molecular characterization of *Brucella* strains isolated from marine mammals. Journal of Clinical Microbiology. 2000;**38**:1258

[7] Mosayebi Z, Movahedian AH, Ghayomi A, Kazemi B. Congenital brucellosis in a preterm neonate. Indian Pediatrics. 2005;**42**:599-601

[8] Imani R, Shamsipoor E, Khadivi R. Congenital brucellosis in an infant. Iranian Journal of Clinical Infectious Diseases. 2007;**2**(1):29-31

[9] Carbajo-Ferreira AJ, Ochoa-Sangrador C, Canut-Blasco A, Castano-Garcia MT. Neonatal brucellosis. The Pediatric Infectious Disease Journal. 1995;**14**:406-407

[10] Singer R, Amitai Y, Geist M, et al. Neonatal brucellosis possibly transmitted during delivery. Lancet. 1991;**338**:127-128

[11] Whatmore AM, Davison N, Cloeckaert A, et al. *Brucella papionis* sp. nov., isolated from baboons (*Papio* spp.). International Journal of Systematic and Evolutionary Microbiology. 2014;**64**:4120

[12] Chheda S, Lopez SM, Sanderson EP. Congenital brucellosis in a premature infant. The Pediatric Infectious Disease Journal. 1997;**16**:81-83

[13] Shamo'on H, Izzat M. Congenital brucellosis. The Pediatric Infectious Disease Journal. 1999;**18**:1110-1111

[14] Giannacopoulos I, Eliopoulou MI, Ziambaras T, Papanastasiou DA. Transplacentally transmitted congenital brucellosis due to *Brucella abortus*. The Journal of Infection. 2002;**45**:209-210

[15] Ruben B, Band JD, Wong P, Colville J. Person to person transmission of *Brucella melitensis*. Lancet. 1991;**337**:14-15

[16] Koklu E, Buyukkayhan D, Akcakus M, Kurtoglu S, Koklu S, Gunes T. Brucellosis with pulmonary involvement in a premature infant. Annals of Tropical Paediatrics. 2006;**26**:367-370

[17] Sarafidis K, Agakidis C, Diamanti E, Karantaglis N, Roilides E. Congenital brucellosis: A rare cause of respiratory

distress in neonates. American Journal of Perinatology. 2007;**24**:409-412

[18] Lubani MM, Dudin KI, Sharda DC, et al. Neonatal brucellosis. European Journal of Pediatrics. 1988;**147**:520-522

[19] Poulou A, Markou F, Xipolitos I, Skandalakis PN. A rare case of *Brucella melitensis* infection in an obstetrician during the delivery of a transplacentally infected infant. The Journal of Infection. 2006;**9**:39-41

[20] Wood EE. Brucellosis as a hazard of blood transfusion. British Medical Journal. 1995;**1**:27-28

[21] Ertem M, Kurekci AE, Aysev D, Unal E, Ikinciogullari A. Brucellosis transmitted by bone marrow transplantation. Bone Marrow Transplantation. 2000;**26**:225-226

[22] Naparstek E, Block CS, Slavin S. Transmission of brucellosis by bone marrow transplantation. Lancet. 1983;**1**:574-575

[23] Palanduz A, Palanduz S, Guler K, Guler N. Brucellosis in a mother and her young infant: Probable transmission by breast milk. International Journal of Infectious Diseases. 2000;**4**:55-56

[24] Lubani M, Sharda D, Helin I. Probable transmission of brucellosis from breast milk to a newborn. Tropical and Geographical Medicine. 1988;**40**:151-152

[25] Celebi G, Kulah C, Kilic S, Ustundag G. Asymptomatic *Brucella* bacteraemia and isolation of *Brucella melitensis* biovar 3 from human breast milk. Scandinavian Journal of Infectious Diseases. 2007;**39**:205-208

[26] Lindquist D, Chu MC, Probert WWS. *Francisella* and *Brucella*. In: Murray PR, Baron EJO, Jorgensen JH, et al., editors. Manual of Clinical Microbiology. 9th ed. Washington, DC: ASM Press; 2007. p. 824

[27] Celli J. The changing nature of the *Brucella*-containing vacuole. Cellular Microbiology. 2015;**17**(7):951-958. DOI: 10.1111/cmi.12452

[28] Jahans KL, Foster G, Broughton ES. The characterisation of *Brucella* strains isolated from marine mammals. Veterinary Microbiology. 1997;**57**:373

[29] Bricker BJ, Halling SM. Differentiation of *Brucella abortus* bv 1,2, and 4, *Brucella melitensis*, *Brucella ovis* and *Brucella suis* bv. 1 by PCR. Journal of Clinical Microbiology. 1994;**32**:2660

[30] Alton GG, Jones LM, Angus RD, Verger JM. Techniques for the Brucellosis Laboratory. Paris: Institute National de la recherche Agronomique; 1988

[31] Muleme M, Mugabi R. "Brucellosis Outbreak Investigations". Sakran et al; 2006

[32] Pappas G, Akritidis N, Bosilkovski M, Tsianos E. Brucellosis. The New England Journal of Medicine. 2005;**352**:2325

[33] Al Dahouk S, Nöckler K. Implications of laboratory diagnosis on brucellosis therapy. Expert Review of Anti-Infective Therapy. 2011;**9**:833

[34] Brown PJB, De Pedro MA, Kysela DT, Van Der Henst C, Kim J, De Bolle X, et al. Polar growth in the alphaproteobacterial order *Rhizobiales*. Proceedings of the National Academy of Sciences. 2012;**109**(5):697-701

[35] Halling SM, Peterson-Burch BD, Bricker BJ, et al. Completion of the genome sequence of *Brucella abortus* and comparison to the highly similar

genomes of *Brucella melitensis* and *Brucella suis*. Journal of Bacteriology. 2005;**187**:2715

[36] Sohn AH, Probert WS, Glaser CA, et al. Human neurobrucellosis with intracerebral granuloma caused by a marine mammal *Brucella* spp. Emerging Infectious Diseases. 2003;**9**:485

[37] McDonald WL, Jamaludin R, Mackereth G, et al. Characterization of a *Brucella* sp. strain as a marine-mammal type despite isolation from a patient with spinal osteomyelitis in New Zealand. Journal of Clinical Microbiology. 2006;**44**:4363

[38] Centers for Disease Control and Prevention (CDC). Human exposures to marine *Brucella* isolated from a harbor porpoise: Maine, 2012. MMWR. Morbidity and Mortality Weekly Report. 2012;**61**:461

[39] Pappas G. The changing *Brucella* ecology: Novel reservoirs, new threats. International Journal of Antimicrobial Agents. 2010;**36**(Suppl 1):S8

[40] Scholz HC, Revilla-Fernández S, Al Dahouk S, et al. *Brucella vulpis* sp. nov., isolated from mandibular lymph nodes of red foxes (*Vulpes vulpes*). International Journal of Systematic and Evolutionary Microbiology. 2016;**66**:2090

[41] DelVecchio VG, Kapatral V, Redkar RJ, et al. The genome sequence of the facultative intracellular pathogen *Brucella melitensis*. Proceedings of the National Academy of Sciences of the United States of America. 2002;**99**:443

[42] Paulsen IT, Seshadri R, Nelson KE, et al. The *Brucella suis* genome reveals fundamental similarities between animal and plant pathogens and symbionts. Proceedings of the National Academy of Sciences of the United States of America. 2002;**99**:13148

[43] Corbel MJ. Brucellosis: An overview. Emerging Infectious Diseases. 1997;**3**:213.27

[44] Al-Eissa Y, Al-Mofada S. Congenital brucellosis. The Pediatric Infectious Disease Journal. 1992;**11**:667-671

[45] Vilchez G, Espinoza M, D'Onadio G, Saona P, et al. Brucellosis in pregnancy: Clinical aspects and obstetric outcomes. International Journal of Infectious Diseases. 2015;**38**:95-100

[46] Nuri P, Volkan T, Mete E, Ozgur Y. Brucellosis in adolescent, pregnancy—Case report and review of literature [in Polish]. Ginekologia Polska. 2011;**82**:226-229

[47] Al-Tawfiq JA, Memish ZA. Pregnancy associated brucellosis. Recent Patents on Anti-Infective Drug Discovery. 2013;**8**:47-50

[48] Al-Anazi K, Al-Jasser A. Brucellosis: A global re-emerging zoonosis history, epidemiology, microbiology, immunology and genetics. In: Mascellino MT, editor. Bacterial and Mycotic Infections in Immunocompromised Hosts; Clinical and Microbiological, Aspects. Saudi Arabia: OMICS Group International; 2013. pp. 1-14

[49] Arenas-Gamboa AM, Rossetti CA, Chaki SP, Garcia-Gonzalez DG, et al. Human brucellosis and adverse pregnancy outcomes. Current Tropical Medicine Reports. 2016;**3**:164-172

[50] Gul S, Khan A. Epidemiology and epizootology of brucellosis: A review. Pakistan Veterinary Journal. 2007;**27**:145

[51] Elkiran O, Kocak G, Karakurt C, Kuzucu C. *Brucella* myocarditis in a 3-month-old: Probable transplacental transmission. Annals of Tropical Paediatrics. 2010;**30**:225-228

[52] Drutz JE. Brucellosis of the central nervous system. A case report of an infected infant. La Clinica Pediatrica. 1989;**28**:476-478

[53] Dogan DG, Aslan M, Menekse E, Yakinci C. Congenital brucellosis: Case report. Annals of Tropical Paediatrics. 2010;**30**:229-231

[54] Yagupsky P. Neonatal brucellosis: Rare and preventable. Annals of Tropical Paediatrics. 2010;**30**:177-179

[55] Tsolia M, Drakonaki S, Messaritaki A, Farmakakis T, Kostaki M, Tsapra H, et al. Clinical features, complications and treatment outcome of childhood brucellosis in central Greece. The Journal of Infection. 2002;**44**:257-262

[56] Khuri-Bulos NA, Daoud AH, Azab SM. Treatment of childhood brucellosis: Results of prospective trial on 113 children. The Pediatric Infectious Disease Journal. 1993;**12**:377-383

Chapter 5

Update of Antibiotic Therapy of Brucellosis

Sara Consuelo Arias Villate and Julio Cesar García Casallas

Abstract

Currently, the only option for treating brucellosis is antibiotics especially to prevent complications. In this chapter, we want to talk about the drug therapy in brucellosis and the update of these therapies in the last years. Also, we will expose the principal antibiotics in brucellosis such as doxycycline, rifampin, streptomycin, cotrimoxazole (TMP/SMX), and gentamicin by talking about each one of their mechanism of action, pharmacokinetics, administration, risk assessment, adverse effects, and principal drug interactions. Furthermore, we will add the evidence of efficacy therapy in monotherapy or combinate therapy based on the evidence.

Keywords: brucellosis, aminoglycoside, doxycycline, rifampin, treatment

1. Introduction

Brucellosis is a zoonotic disease that can affect humans around the world, and it can affect any organ system. About the treatment, it is characterized to be prolonged therapy with a concomitant use of at least two or three antibiotics at different administration routes. The antibiotics have some special indications for administration, interactions, and risk assessment to prevent adverse reactions. That is why we will expose the principal antibiotics in brucellosis treatment based on the last evidence.

2. Antibiotic treatment

The principal objective of the treatment in brucellosis is to control the disease, prevent complications, relapse, and unfavorable outcomes. In the context of a zoonotic infection, the goal of its management is an appropriate antibiotic therapy with a prolonged duration of treatment, nevertheless the most effective antibiotic and treatment durations are unclear. Also, there are some limitations to choose the best treatment because of the need to choose antibiotics that act intracellularly and to prevent relapses with a prolonged therapy that can lead to increase the adverse effects of the drugs [1].

Furthermore, the monotherapy for brucellosis has been considered inadequate due to unacceptably high relapse rates, now we present possible treatment schemes [2, 3].

Uncomplicated brucellosis: (defined by not having focal disease like spondylitis, neurobrucellosis or endocarditis, and adults or > 30 kg):

- Doxycycline 100 mg orally twice daily for 6 weeks, plus streptomycin 1 g intramuscularly one daily for the first 14–21 days (or gentamicin 5 mg/kg for 5–14 days) [1, 2, 4].

- Doxycycline 100 mg orally twice daily plus rifampin 600–900 mg (15 mg/kg) orally one daily for 6 weeks [1, 3].
- Consider triple therapy with addition of amikacin (intramuscularly twice a day for 7 days) to relief symptoms more rapid.

Alternative agents: (they may be useful in the setting of drug resistance, allergy, antimicrobial toxicity or relapse in combination with doxycycline or rifampin)

- Ciprofloxacin 500 mg twice daily or ofloxacin 200 mg twice daily [5, 6].
- Trimethoprim-sulfamethoxazole (TMP-SMX) one double-strength tablet twice a day.

Focal disease: spondylitis, neurobrucellosis, endocarditis, or localized suppurative lesions (it requires longer courses of therapy at least 12 weeks):

- Spondylitis
  - Doxycycline 100 mg orally twice daily for 12 weeks plus streptomycin 1 g intramuscularly once daily for the first 14–21 days [7].
  - Alternative: doxycycline 100 mg orally twice daily plus rifampin 600–900 mg (15 mg/kg) once daily for 12 weeks.
  - Surgery in the context of spinal instability, persistence or progression of neurological deficit or localizes abscess epidural or paravertebral [8].
- Neurobrucellosis
  - Doxycycline, rifampin, and ceftriaxone or TMP-SMX.
  - Corticosteroids may be appropriate in the setting of neurobrucellosis complicated by iritis, papilledema, myelopathy, polyneuropathy, or cranial nerve palsies.
- Endocarditis
  - Doxycycline plus rifampin 300 mg every 12 h and gentamycin 5 mg/kg each day, the duration of therapy is uncertain usually for 6 weeks to 6 months [9].
  - Surgery: valve replacement.

Pregnant women: [2, 10].

- Limited data.
- Rifampin 900 mg once daily, with or without TMP-SMV (one double-strength tablet twice a day) for 6 weeks or rifampin with ceftriaxone.

Children

- Uncomplicated brucellosis

- (<8 years of age): oral TMP-SMX [10 mg/kg per day TMP (maximum 480 mg/day) and 50 mg/kg per day SMX (maximum 2.4 g/day) by mouth divided into two doses] daily plus rifampin [15–20 mg/kg per day by mouth (maximum 900 mg/day) divided in one or two doses] (or gentamycin 5 mg/kg IV daily for 7 days) for 6 weeks [10–12].
- (>8 years of age): oral doxycycline [2–4 mg/kg per day by mouth (maximum 200 mg/day) divided into two doses] or tetracycline [30–40 mg/kg per day by mouth (maximum 2 g/day) divided into four doses] plus rifampin for 6 weeks [11].

- Osteoarticular disease, neurobrucellosis, or endocarditis
  - <8 years of age: oral TMP-SMX for at least 6 weeks plus parenteral aminoglycoside [gentamicin (5 mg/kg per day parenterally divided into one to three doses) or streptomycin (20–40 mg/kg per day (maximum dose 1 g/day) parenterally divided in two doses)] for the first 14 days of therapy.
  - >8 years of age: oral doxycycline or tetracycline for at least 6 weeks, plus parenteral aminoglycoside (gentamicin or streptomycin) for the first 14 days of therapy.

2.1 Doxycycline

2.1.1 Mechanism of action

It belongs to the group of tetracyclines that are a series of derivatives of basic four-ring structure. Doxycycline inhibits bacterial protein synthesis by binding to the 30S bacterial ribosome and blocking the access of aminoacyl tRNA to the A (acceptor) site on the mRNA-ribosome complex and inhibits protein synthesis [13].

2.1.2 Antimicrobial activity

Doxycycline is a bacteriostatic antibiotic with activity against *Streptococcus pneumoniae* and *H. influenzae* and excellent activity against atypical pathogens such as *Mycoplasma* and *Chlamydophila pneumoniae*, methicillin-resistant *Staphylococcus aureus* and methicillin-susceptible *Staphylococcus aureus*, *Bacillus anthracis*, and *Listeria monocytogenes* and most strains of *Brucella* are susceptible. Some species such as *Pseudomonas aeruginosa* are resistant [13, 14].

2.1.3 Pharmacokinetics

See **Table 1**.

2.1.4 Administration

- Oral: administer with meals to decrease gastrointestinal (GI) discomfort. Administer capsules and tablets with a considerable amount of water and have patient sit up for at least 30 minutes to reduce esophageal irritation. Oral administration is preferable unless patient has significant nausea and vomiting [13].
- IV: infuse prolonged over 1–4 hours to prevent thrombophlebitis.

Absorption	Oral: almost completely absorbed from the gastrointestinal tract (GI) (90–100%), plasma concentration may be reduced 20% by high-fat meal or milk Time to peak serum: oral: 2–4 hours
Distribution	Widely distributed into tissues and fluids including synovial, pleural, prostatic, seminal fluids and bronchial secretions, saliva, aqueous humor Poor cerebrospinal fluid penetration Protein binding: >90% Distribution volume Bioavailability: reduced at high pH
Metabolism	Not hepatic, partially inactivated in GI tract by chelate formation
Elimination	Half-time elimination: 18–22 hours, end-stage renal disease: 18–25 hours Excretion: feces (30%); urine (23–40%)

Table 1.
Pharmacokinetics parameters of doxycycline [13].

2.1.5 Risk assessment

When therapy of doxycycline needs to be used in prolonged therapy, some parameters need to be taken to prevent some of the adverse effects: complete blood count (CBC), renal and liver function tests periodically, during therapy [13].

2.1.6 Adverse effects

- Gastrointestinal: it can produce GI irritation especially after oral administration (epigastric burning, abdominal discomfort, nausea, vomiting and diarrhea). To prevent this, the patient should take oral formulations with a glass full of water, administration on an empty stomach is generally not recommended [14].

- Photosensitivity: it may produce photosensitivity reactions in treated individuals exposed to sunlight. The patient needs to use skin protection and avoid prolonged exposure to sunlight and ultraviolet light [14].

- Hepatotoxicity: rarely occurs during the treatment. If patient became symptomatic, assess liver function tests, and discontinue drug [14].

- Hypersensitivity syndromes: severe skin reactions have been reported. Discontinue therapy for serious hypersensitivity reactions.

- Superinfection: prolonged use may result in fungal or bacterial superinfection like pseudomembranous colitis.

- Tissue hyperpigmentation: may induce hyperpigmentation in many organs: nails, bone, skin, eyes, thyroid, oral cavity (permanent brown discoloration of the teeth in children <8 years or in children from pregnant women in their last half of pregnancy), and sclerae, most dependently of time and chronic use [15].

2.1.7 Principal drug interactions

See **Table 2**.

Drug	Risk rating	Interaction	Mechanism	Management
Antacids (aluminum hydroxide, calcium carbonate, magnesium carbonate, sodium bicarbonate)	Consider therapy modification	Antacids may decrease the absorption of doxycycline	Formation of chelates between antibiotic and antacids that reduces absorption from the GI tract [16]	Separate administration of both by a few hours when possible Monitor for decreased therapeutic effects of antibiotic [17]
Barbiturates	Consider therapy modification	Barbiturates may decrease the serum concentration of doxycycline	Uncertain. Induction of doxycycline metabolism or excretion by the barbiturates [18]	Monitor decreased therapeutic effects of antibiotic if used concurrently with a barbiturate
Aspirin	Monitor therapy	Aspirin may decrease the serum concentration of doxycycline	Buffered aspirin contains antacids that alkaline environment may also reduce absorption [19]	Administer doxycycline at least 2 hours before or 6 hours after aspirin ingestion
Rifampin	Monitor therapy	Rifampin may decrease the serum concentration of doxycycline	Unknown. Rifampin induction of doxycycline metabolism and/ or excretion [20]	Monitor closely for reduced doxycycline response in patients receiving rifampin

Table 2.
Principal drug interactions of doxycycline.

2.1.8 Important

- Tetracyclines are inexpensive, widely available, and poor associated with side effects, and also it have proven safe in all age groups [21].
- The doxycycline-streptomycin regimen is considered the first line and has been proven to be more effective than doxycycline-rifampin in some studies [4, 22].
- Do not administer to children <8 years of age due to permanent discoloration of teeth, retardation of skeletal development, and bone growth; more common with long-term use, but may be observed with repeated, short courses [12, 23].

2.2 Streptomycin

2.2.1 Mechanism of action

It is an aminoglycoside antibiotic bactericidal. Aminoglycosides diffuse through aqueous channels formed by porin proteins in the outer membrane of Gram-negative bacteria to enter to the periplasmic space, and its transport across the cytoplasmic membrane depends on an electrical gradient coupled to electron transport to drive permeation of these antibiotics. That is why they are not used in anaerobic environments of abscess. Once streptomycin is inside the cell, it binds to the 30S ribosomal subunit and interferes with protein synthesis by causing misreading and premature termination of mRNA translation, and the resulting aberrant proteins may be inserted into the cell membrane altering permeability [24–26].

2.2.2 Antimicrobial activity

It is less active than other members of the class against aerobic Gram-negative, and it is used for the treatment of unusual infections and in combination with other antimicrobial agents. The inhibitory activity of aminoglycosides persists after the serum concentration has fallen below de minimum inhibitory concentration (MIC), and it is known as the post antibiotic effect and it improves the efficacy of high-dose extended-interval dosing regimens for aminoglycoside. It is used for the treatment of tuberculosis, tularemia, severe *M. avium* complex, brucellosis, and enterococcal endocarditis in combination with other drugs [24, 27].

2.2.3 Pharmacokinetics

See **Table 3**.

Absorption	Oral: poorly absorbed, IM: well absorbed Time to peak IM: 1–2 hours
Distribution	Into most body tissues and fluids except the brain and adipose tissue (because of their polar nature) Protein binding: 34% Volume of distribution (Vd): 260 mL/kg
Metabolism	None known
Excretion	Half-time elimination: adults: 2–4, 7 hours, prolonged with renal impairment Urine: 29–89% as unchanged drug Bile, saliva, sweat and tears: (1%)

Table 3.
Pharmacokinetic parameters of streptomycin [24, 28].

2.2.4 Administration

Streptomycin may be administered by deep intramuscular injection into large muscle mass, rotate injection sites (it may be painful with a hot tender mass developing at the site injection) or intravenously (after dilution in admixture, infuse over 30–60 minutes). High-dose, extended-interval administration is the preferred administration of aminoglycosides because of less toxic effect than divided doses [24, 27].

2.2.5 Risk assessment

It is important to monitor hearing tests (baseline and periodic audiograms), BUN, creatinine, and serum drug concentrations should be monitored in all patients:

- Therapeutic peak: 20–30 mcg/mL [25].

2.2.6 Adverse effects

- Ototoxicity: aminoglycoside induces ototoxicity irreversible, bilateral, high-frequency hearing loss or vestibular hypofunction. It has been seen degeneration of hair cells and neurons in the cochlea and accumulation in the perilymph and endolymph at high antibiotic concentration in plasma. The initial symptoms such as high-pitched tinnitus, nausea, vomiting, and difficulty in equilibrium may be reversible, so it should be monitored carefully for ototoxicity [24].

- Nephrotoxicity: it is because the accumulation and retention of aminoglycoside in the proximal tubular cells and the initial manifestations of damage at this site are mild proteinuria and hyaline and granular casts, and also the glomerular filtration rate is reduced after several additional days [24].

2.2.7 Principal drug interactions

See **Table 4**.

Drug	Risk rating	Interaction	Mechanism	Management
Colistimethate	Consider therapy modification	Aminoglycosides may enhance the nephrotoxic and neuromuscular-blocking effect of colistimethate	Additive nephrotoxic effects Alteration in membrane permeability that leads to cellular lysis by colistimethate [29, 30]	This combination should be avoided, if they must be used together to monitor patients' renal and neuromuscular function
Penicillins	Consider therapy modification	Penicillins may decrease the serum concentration of aminoglycosides	Inactivation of aminoglycosides by extended spectrum penicillins, especially in renal dysfunction [31, 32]	Monitor serum aminoglycoside concentration, and do not administer dose together through the same IV line

Table 4.
Principal drug interactions of streptomycin.

2.2.8 Important

- Streptomycin is not available always in some regions and it is administered only intramuscularly or intravenously, so it is a disadvantage [2].

- Gentamicin has replaced streptomycin for some indications because the toxicity of gentamicin is renal and mostly reversible although streptomycin is most vestibular compromise and irreversible [24].

2.3 Gentamicin

2.3.1 Mechanism of action

Gentamicin is a bactericidal aminoglycoside. It binds to the 30S ribosomal subunit and interferes with initiation of protein synthesis causing misreading of mRNA, premature termination of translation, and incomplete synthesized protein, creating nonfunctional proteins [24, 33].

2.3.2 Antimicrobial activity

Gram-negative bacteria such as *Pseudomonas aeruginosa*, *Proteus* species, *Escherichia coli*, *Klebsiella* species, *Enterobacter* species, *Serratia*, *Citrobacter*, and *Staphylococcus* species [24].

2.3.3 Pharmacokinetics

See **Table 5**.

Absorption	Intramuscular: rapid and complete Oral: poorly absorbed Time to peak: IM 30–90 minutes; IV: 30 minutes after 30-minute infusion
Distribution	Primarily into extracellular fluid, renal cortex. Poor penetration in cerebrospinal fluid (CSF) and ocular tissues Vd: children: 0.35 L/kg; adults: 0.2–0.3 L/kg Protein binding: <30%
Metabolism	Minimal metabolism
Excretion	Half-life elimination: adults 2 hours, renal failure: 41–24 hours Urine: >70% as unchanged drug Clearance is decreased in renal impairment

Table 5.
Pharmacokinetic parameters of gentamicin [24, 34, 35].

2.3.4 Administration

- IM: it should be administered by deep IM route.
- IV: infuse over 30–120 minutes [27].

2.3.5 Risk assessment

During therapy with gentamicin, you should monitor parameters like: urinalysis, urine output, BUN, serum creatinine, plasma gentamicin levels (before and after the third dose), hearing tests before, during and after treatment especially in prolonged therapy [36, 37].

- Therapeutic peak: 5 and 12 μg/mL [36, 37].

2.3.6 Adverse effects

- Nephrotoxicity: usual risk factors include preexisting renal impairment, concomitant nephrotoxicity drugs, advanced age, and dehydration. If nephrotoxicity occurs, it is better to discontinue therapy because the renal damage is usually reversible [24, 38].
- Ototoxicity: use with caution in patients with preexisting vertigo, tinnitus or hearing loss [24, 38].
- Neuromuscular blockade: aminoglycosides may inhibit prejunctional release of acetylcholine reducing postsynaptic sensitivity to the transmitter, and this reaction can follow intravenous, intramuscular or even oral administration of this antibiotics, especially with concomitant use of anesthesia and other neuromuscular blocking agents. It can be reversed by intravenous administration of calcium salt [24].

2.3.7 Principal drug interactions

See **Table 6**.

Drug	Risk rating	Interaction	Mechanism	Management
Amphotericin B	Monitor therapy	Amphotericin B may enhance the nephrotoxic effect of aminoglycosides	Unknown. Probably synergism [39]	Monitor renal function
Bisphosphonate derivatives	Monitor therapy	Aminoglycosides may enhance the hypocalcemic effect of bisphosphonate derivates [40]	Association of aminoglycosides with hypocalcemia, probably inhibition of the activity of the parathyroid glands reducing parathyroid hormone production [40, 41]	Monitor serum calcium, serum magnesium and serum creatinine and renal function during concomitant use
Furosemide, bumetanide, torsemide (loop diuretics)	Monitor therapy	Diuretics may enhance nephrotoxicity and ototoxicity of aminoglycosides	Uncertain. Damage in proximal tubular cells and decrease glomerular filtration rate. [42, 43]	Monitor toxic effects or avoid concomitant use except in life-threatening situations

Table 6.
Principal drug interactions of gentamicin.

2.4 Rifampin

2.4.1 Mechanism of action

Rifampin is a bactericidal drug that kills cell growing and it binds to the beta subunit of DNA-dependent RNA polymerase (rpoB) to form a drug-enzyme complex blocking the chain formation in RNA transcription [44].

2.4.2 Antimicrobial activity

It inhibits most Gram-positive bacteria and Gram-negative microorganisms such as *Escherichia coli*, *Pseudomonas*, *Proteus*, and *Klebsiella*, and also it is active again *Neisseria meningitidis*, *Haemophilus influenzae*, and *Mycobacterium tuberculosis* [44].

2.4.3 Pharmacokinetics

See **Table 7**.

Absorption	Oral: well absorbed (bioavailability 68%). Food may delay or reduce peak by one-third. It should be taken on an empty stomach Time to peak serum: oral: 2–4 hours
Distribution	Good penetration into many tissues and crosses CSF Vd: 53 L/kg Protein binding: 80%
Metabolism	Microsomal B-esterases and cholinesterases. Also, 85% liver metabolism (potently induction CYP 1A2, 2C9, 2C19 and 3A4) and enterohepatic recirculation
Excretion	Half-life elimination: 3–4 hours, prolonged with hepatic impairment feces (60%) and urine (30%) as unchanged drug

Table 7.
Pharmacokinetic parameters of rifampin [34, 44–46].

2.4.4 Administration

- IV: administer IV preparation by slow infusion rate IV over 30 minutes to 3 hours, monitor administration to prevent extravasation.

- Do not administer IM or SC.

- Oral: administer on an empty stomach with a glass of water to increase absorption [44].

2.4.5 Risk assessment

During the therapy with rifampin, it should be monitored with periodical liver function test, CBC, and therapeutic drug monitoring of rifampin [47].

2.4.6 Adverse effects

- Hypersensitivity reactions: cases of severe cutaneous adverse reactions like Stevens-Johnson syndrome, toxic epidermal necrolysis, and drug reaction with eosinophilia. It is mediated by hypersensitivity type I (IgE). It requires discontinue of therapy and management of the symptoms [48].

- Flu-like syndrome: symptoms of fever, chills, headache related with the use of oral rifampin. It is related with regimens of >600 mg once or twice weekly, and it resolves spontaneously. Flu-like syndrome is mediated by hypersensitivity type III (antibodies against rifampicin IgM that produce immunocomplex) [48, 49].

- Hematologic effects: it may cause thrombocytopenia, leukopenia, or anemia. The platelets are damaged by complement activation following the formation of drug-antibody complex [48, 50].

- Hepatotoxicity: it may cause hepatic dysfunction especially if it is used with other hepatotoxic agents [44].

2.4.7 Principal drug interactions

Most of the interactions of rifampin are because it is a strong inducer of CYP3A4 and CYP2C19, moderate inducer of CYP2C8 and CYP2C9, and P-glycoprotein inducer (**Table 8**) [51].

2.4.8 Important

- In children, pregnant or lactating women rifampin should not be used except where tetracyclines are contraindicated or when there are limitations on the use of streptomycin or gentamicin and it should not be used alone [1, 6, 9].

- It can be an alternative treatment for doxycycline or aminoglycosides, but the use of rifampin should be restricted in endemic areas of tuberculosis because monotherapy with rifampin can lead to the selection of resistant *Mycobacterium tuberculosis* strains [1, 3, 6, 9].

Drug	Risk rating	Interaction	Mechanism	Management
Apixaban	Avoid combination	Rifampin is a strong inducer CYP3A4 and may decrease the serum concentration of apixaban	Induction of the CYP3A4-mediated metabolism of apixaban [52]	Avoid concurrent use
Esomeprazole	Avoid combination	Rifampin may decrease the serum concentration of esomeprazole	Rifampin induction of CYP3A4- and CYP2C19-mediated esomeprazole metabolism [53]	Avoid concomitant use
Risperidone	Consider therapy modification	Rifampin is a CYP3A4 inducer that may decrease the serum concentration of risperidone [46]	Unknown. Enzyme-inducing drugs may decrease risperidone [54]	Consider increasing the dose of oral risperidone (no more than double the original dose) if a CYP3A4 inducer is initiated

Table 8.
Principal drug interactions of rifampin [55].

2.5 Ciprofloxacin

2.5.1 Mechanism of action

The fluoroquinolones inhibit two bacterial enzymes: DNA gyrase (in many Gram-negative bacteria) and topoisomerase IV (in many Gram-positive bacteria) blocking the DNA bacterial replication. This action results in damage of bacterial DNA and cell death being bactericidal agents [56, 57].

2.5.2 Antimicrobial activity

It is a bactericidal agent against *Proteus*, *E. coli*, *Klebsiella*, *Salmonella*, *Shigella*, *Enterobacter*, and *Campylobacter* [56].

2.5.3 Pharmacokinetics

See **Table 9**.

Absorption	Oral: well absorbed Bioavailability: 70%. Avoid taking with most antacids and milk
Distribution	Widely distributed in kidneys, gallbladder, liver, lungs, gynecological tissue, and prostatic tissue Protein binding: 20–40% Vd: 2.1–2.7 L/kg
Metabolism	Poor hepatic metabolism and forms 4 metabolites, inhibitor of CYP1A2
Excretion	Half-life elimination: children: 4–5 hours and adults: 3–5 hours, prolonged in older adults and in renal impairment Urine 50% as unchanged drug), feces (15%)

Table 9.
Pharmacokinetic parameters of ciprofloxacin [55, 56].

2.5.4 Administration

- Oral: administer with food to minimize GI symptoms, avoid antacid use, milk, yogurt or calcium-fortified juices alone.
- IV: administer by slow IV infusion over 60 minutes [56].

2.5.5 Risk assessment

During the treatment with ciprofloxacin parameters like: CBC, renal and hepatic function, signs and symptoms of tendonitis should be monitored [56].

2.5.6 Adverse effects

- Gastrointestinal: nausea, vomiting, and abdominal discomfort [56].
- Neurologic: headache and dizziness, peripheral neuropathy, it can occur at any time during treatment and can last for months to years after finishing the treatment [58].
- Musculoskeletal: tendon rupture or tendinitis usually of the Achilles tendon, arthralgias, and join pain are reported, especially in ancient people and patients taking corticosteroids [59, 60].
- QT interval prolongation and arrhythmia: it may be produced by inhibition of potassium channels encoded by the KCNH2 gene (HERG gene). Ciprofloxacin use should be avoided in patients with a history of QT prolongation, torsade de pointes, uncorrected hypokalemia, cardiac disease or concomitant use of other medications that prolong the QT interval [56, 61].

2.5.7 Principal drug interactions

See **Table 10**.

Drug	Risk rating	Interaction	Mechanism	Management
Antacids, multivitamins and minerals like folate and iron	Consider therapy modification	Antacids may decrease the absorption of quinolones	The carbonyl functional groups on the antibiotic forms a chelate with the cations of the antacid resulting in inactive antimicrobials [62, 63]	Avoid concurrent administration of quinolones and antacids or quinolones should be administered at least 2 hours before or 2 hours after antacids or 6 hours after multivitamins
Theophylline	Consider therapy modification	Quinolones may decrease the metabolism of theophylline	Quinolone inhibition of CYP1A2 and CYP3A4 isoenzymes limiting the metabolism of theophylline [64, 65]	Consider a reduction in the dosage of theophylline (25–50%) during the concurrent use to minimize the theophylline toxicity

Table 10.
Principal drug interactions of ciprofloxacin.

2.5.8 Important

- It may be useful in the setting of drug resistance, antimicrobial toxicity, and some cases of relapse.

2.6 Trimethoprim-sulfamethoxazole (TMP/SMX)

2.6.1 Mechanism of action

The combination of trimethoprim with sulfamethoxazole enhances the effectivity and synergist antimicrobial activity. TMP inhibits bacterial dihydrofolate reductase preventing the formation of tetrahydrofolic acid, and SMX is a structural analog of the para-aminobenzoic acid (PABA), and it binds to the dihydropteroate synthetase and competes with PABA to inhibit the synthesis of dihydrofolic acid [56, 66].

2.6.2 Antimicrobial activity

The antibacterial spectrum is most *S. pneumoniae*, *S. aureus*, and *Staphylococcus epidermidis*, some *E. coli* according to the geographic region, *Proteus mirabilis*, *Klebsiella*, *Enterobacter*, also *Brucella abortus* [56].

2.6.3 Pharmacokinetics

See **Table 11**.

Absorption	Oral: rapid 90–100%, TMP is absorbed more rapidly than sulfamethoxazole, bioavailability of 85%
Distribution	Good penetration in middle ear fluid, sputum, vaginal fluid, and bronchial secretions Vd: adults: 1.3 L/kg Protein binding: SMX 70%, TMP 44%
Metabolism	Hepatic, SMX via CYP2C9 and also conjugated with glucuronide; TMP to oxide and hydroxy derivatives
Excretion	Half time elimination: TMP: children 3.7–5.5 hours and adults: 6–11 hours. SMX 9–12 hours Both excreted in urine as metabolites and unchanged drug

Table 11.
Pharmacokinetic parameters of TMP/SMX [56].

2.6.4 Administration

- Oral: administer without regard to meals and a lot of water.
- IV: infuse over 60–90 minutes, and it is not administered by IM injection [56].

2.6.5 Risk assessment

Some monitoring parameters during the treatment are CBC, serum potassium, creatinine, and BUN [56].

2.6.6 Adverse effects

- Blood dyscrasias: agranulocytosis, aplastic anemia, leukopenia, or thrombocytopenia because of the margin between toxicity for bacteria and humans related with folate deficient [67].
- Neurologic effects: it is associated with adverse neurologic events like aseptic meningitis, tremor, delirium because TMP/SMX crosses the blood-brain barrier [67].
- Dermatologic reactions: severe reactions including Stevens-Johnson syndrome produced by immune-mediated idiosyncratic reactions associated with reactive metabolite leading to drug-specific antibodies [67].
- Hyperkalemia: it is produced because of the TMP similar structure to potassium-sparing diuretics. Potential risk factors include renal impairment, older age, and concomitant use of medications causing or exacerbating hyperkalemia [56].

2.6.7 Principal drug interactions

See **Table 12**.

Drug	Risk rating	Interaction	Mechanism	Management
Phenytoin	Consider therapy modification	TMP/SMX may increase the serum concentration of phenytoin	TMP inhibition of CYP2C8 and CYP2C9-mediated phenytoin metabolism [68]	Consider alternatives to this combination when possible
Warfarin	Consider therapy modification	TMP/SMX may enhance the anticoagulant effect of vitamin K antagonists	Multifactorial. Sulfonamide displacement of warfarin from protein binding sites, reductions in GI flora responsible for production of vitamin K [69, 70]	Monitor toxic effects of warfarin. Consider reducing warfarin dose by 10–20% prior starting the sulfonamide antibiotic and monitoring INR closely [71]

Table 12.
Principal drug interactions of TMP/SMX.

2.6.8 Important

- TMP-SMX may be used as an additional agent in complex cases of focal brucellosis, relapse, or refractory disease [2].
- TMP-SMZ should not be used in pregnancy, either before 13 weeks because of the risk of teratogenic effects or after 36 weeks because of the risk of kernicterus [21].
- It has been a popular choice and it is included in combination regimens around the world, due to its lower cost compared to other antimicrobials being the most cost-effective drug against brucellosis in developing countries [2].
- No alternative anti-brucellosis therapy for children under 8 years old has been reported, but there is a case that had a 2.5 years old patient with brucellosis

with TMP-SMX allergy, they use as an alternative for treatment ciprofloxacin having a good result of the treatment and continue follow up visits, but there are no evidence enough for this treatment, so it is necessary to search for alternative treatment for this patient population [12].

3. Other considerations about treatment

- Doxycycline is the drug of choice in the treatment of brucellosis, but antibiotic susceptibility patterns of *Brucella* appears to vary geographically, that is why tigecycline can be an option for treatment in brucellosis. Tigecycline is a glycylcycline derivate from tetracycline and minocycline. It has demonstrated activity against *Enterobacteriaceae*, Gram-positives, atypical, and anaerobes. It has the lowest minimal inhibitory concentration on in vitro efficacy models, and also it provided the better synergistic activity compared to doxycycline. Tigecycline can be a therapeutic alternative for brucellosis especially in patients in whom conventional antibiotics is contraindicated or limited because of the presence of severe comorbidities or drug-drug interactions, but it should be supported with more clinical studies [72].

- There are some regional experience and some different treatments that differs according the regional experiences but here are some considerations:

    - The World Health Organization (WHO) recommends the use of doxycycline for 6 weeks combined with rifampicin for 6 weeks, or streptomycin for 2–3 weeks, but this regimen has not been universally used in clinical practice. Even this fact it remains unclear what is the best regimen to be used and more clinical studies are needed in this regard [2].

    - From the comparison of regimens that can be established in randomized clinical trials are: doxycycline and streptomycin vs. doxycycline and rifampicin that favors the first combination in terms of relapse (OR 3.52; CI 95% = 2.14–5.81; $p < 0.001$); doxycycline and streptomycin vs. doxycycline and gentamicin is not statistically significant as regards either relapses (OR = 1.65; CI 95% = 0.53–5.15; $p = 0.386$); doxycycline and rifampicin vs. doxycycline and quinolone favors the first one (OR 3.92; CI 95% = 1.35–11.42; $p = 0.01$) [73].

    - The most effective regimen is combined doxycycline for 45 days with streptomycin for 14 days, in endemic areas where many patients have a mild form of the disease and diagnosis and prescription can be made in the urgency room the used to use gentamycin for the first 5–7 days [4, 73].

    - About the comparison of the efficacy of gentamicin for 5 days plus doxycycline for 8 weeks vs. streptomycin for 2 weeks plus doxycycline for 45 days in human brucellosis, there is a clinical trial that compare the efficacy showing that this treatment is not superior to the standard treatment regimen [74].

    - There are a few studies using doxycycline, rifampicin, and aminoglycosides vs. other regimens in uncomplicated brucellosis with no conclusions on the value of this triple therapy, also some studies were performed only in patients with osteoarticular complications. Another option for triple therapy is doxycycline, rifampin, and amikacin (intramuscularly twice a day for 7 days) that have higher efficacy and more rapid action in terms of relief of symptoms, but it has no significant difference in drug side-effects and disease relapse, thus adding amikacin to the standard treatment regimen seems beneficial [6, 75].

4. Conclusion

In conclusion, there are some antibiotic therapies that are approved for the treatment of brucellosis, and some of them are in prolonged therapy that could affect the adherence of the patient and some of the antibiotics have important recommendations and need to be used in some conditions. Also, they have some parameters that may be monitorable to prevent adverse effects and to improve the outcome of the treatment in all the patients.

Conflict of interest

The authors declare no conflict of interest.

Notes/thanks/other declarations

None.

Appendices and nomenclature

CBC	complete blood count
GI	gastrointestinal
h	hours
IM	intramuscular
IV	intravenous
kg	kilograms
mg	milligrams
MIC	minimum Inhibitory concentration
TMP/SMX	trimethoprim-sulfamethoxazole
Vd	volume of distribution

Author details

Sara Consuelo Arias Villate and Julio Cesar García Casallas*
Evidence-Based Therapeutic Group, Clinical Pharmacology, Universidad de La Sabana, Chia, Colombia

*Address all correspondence to: julio.garcia@unisabana.edu.co

References

[1] Yousefi-Nooraie R, Mortaz-Hejri S, Mehrani M, Sadeghipour P. Antibiotics for treating human brucellosis. Cochrane Database of Systematic Reviews. 2012;**10**:CD007179. DOI: 10.1002/14651858.CD007179.pub2

[2] Ariza J, Bosilkovski M, Cascio A, Colmenero JD, Corbel MJ, Falagas ME, et al. Perspectives for the treatment of brucellosis in the 21st century: The ioannina recommendations. PLoS Medicine. 2007;**4**(12):e317. DOI: 10.1371/journal.pmed.0040317

[3] Tuon FF, Cerchiari N, Cequinel JC, Droppa EEH, Moreira SDR, Costa TP, et al. Guidelines for the management of human brucellosis in the state of Paraná, Brazil. Revista da Sociedade Brasileira de Medicina Tropical. 2017;**50**(4):458-464. DOI: 10.1590/0037-8682-0319-2016

[4] Skalsky K, Yahav D, Bishara J, Pitlik S, Leibovici L, Paul M. Treatment of human brucellosis: Systematic review and meta-analysis of randomised controlled trials. The British Medical Journal. 2008;**336**(7646):701-704. DOI: 10.1136/bmj.39497.500903.25

[5] Falagas ME, Bliziotis IA. Quinolones for treatment of human brucellosis: Critical review of the evidence from microbiological and clinical studies. Antimicrobial Agents and Chemotherapy. 2006;**50**(1):22-33. DOI: 10.1128/AAC.50.1.22-33.2006

[6] Alavi SM, Alavi L. Treatment of brucellosis: A systematic review of studies in recent twenty years. Caspian Journal of Internal Medicine. 2013;**4**(2):636-641

[7] Alp E, Doganay M. Current therapeutic strategy in spinal brucellosis. International Journal of Infectious Diseases. 2008;**12**(6):573-577. DOI: 10.1016/j.ijid.2008.03.014

[8] Alp E, Koc RK, Durak AC, Yildiz O, Aygen B, Sumerkan B, et al. Doxycycline plus streptomycin versus ciprofloxacin plus rifampicin in spinal brucellosis [ISRCTN31053647]. BMC Infectious Diseases. 2006;**6**(1):72. DOI: 10.1186/1471-2334-6-72

[9] Mani SR, Gunasekaran K, Iyyadurai R, Prakash JJ, Veeraraghavan B, Mishra A, et al. Clinical spectrum, susceptibility profile, treatment and outcome of culture-confirmed brucellosis from South India. Indian Journal of Medical Microbiology. 2018;**36**(2):289. DOI: 10.4103/ijmm.IJMM_18_236

[10] Castaño MJ, Navarro E, Solera J. Brucellosis, International Encyclopedia of Public Health. 2nd ed. Academic Press; 2017. pp. 281-295. ISBN: 9780128037089. https://doi.org/10.1016/B978-0-12-803678-5.00041-2

[11] Vollmar P, Zange S, Zöller L, Erkel J, Robert Thoma B. Brucellose. Deutsche Medizinische Wochenschrift. 2016;**141**(14):1014-1018. DOI: 10.1055/s-0042-101723

[12] Teker D, Tanir G, Ozmen S, Teke TA, Keles S, Bostancı I. Treatment of brucellosis in a young child with trimethoprim/sulfamethoxazole anaphylaxis. Journal of Infection and Public Health. 2014;7(6):553-556. DOI: 10.1016/J.JIPH.2014.07.004

[13] MacDougal C. Protein synthesis inhibitors and miscellaneous antibacterial agents. In: Shanahan JF, Lebowitz H, editors. Goodman & Gilman's: The Pharmacological Basis of Therapeutics. 13th ed. United States of America: Access Medicine, McGraw-Hill Medical; 2018

[14] Joshi N, Miller DQ. Doxycycline revisited. Archives of Internal Medicine. 1997;**157**(13):1421-1428

[15] Diseases C on I, Pediatrics of AA. 2015 Report of the Committee on Infectious Diseases Red Book®. 30th ed. 2015

[16] Ogawa R, Echizen H. Clinically significant drug interactions with antacids. Drugs. 2011;**71**(14):1839-1864. DOI: 10.2165/11593990-000000000-00000

[17] Nguyen VX, Nix DE, Gillikin S, Schentag JJ. Effect of oral antacid administration on the pharmacokinetics of intravenous doxycycline. Antimicrobial Agents and Chemotherapy. 1989;**33**(4):434-436

[18] Neuvonen PJ, Penttilä O. Interaction between doxycycline and barbiturates. British Medical Journal. 1974;**1**(5907):535-536

[19] Jaffe JM, Colaizzi JL, Poust RI, McDonald RH. Effect of altered urinarypH on tetracycline and doxycycline excretion in humans. Journal of Pharmacokinetics and Biopharmaceutics. 1973;**1**(4):267-282. DOI: 10.1007/BF01060035

[20] Colmenero JD, Fernández-Gallardo LC, Agúndez JA, Sedeño J, Benítez J, Valverde E. Possible implications of doxycycline-rifampin interaction for treatment of brucellosis. Antimicrobial Agents and Chemotherapy. 1994;**38**(12):2798-2802

[21] Solera J. Update on brucellosis: Therapeutic challenges. International Journal of Antimicrobial Agents. 2010;**36**:S18-S20. DOI: 10.1016/J.IJANTIMICAG.2010.06.015

[22] Solera J, Martínez-Alfaro E, Sáez L. Meta-analysis of the efficacy of the combination of +rifampicin and doxycycline in the treatment of human brucellosis. Medicina Clínica (Barcelona). 1994;**102**(19):731-738

[23] Bukhari EE. Pediatric brucellosis. An update review for the new millennium. Saudi Medical Journal. 2018;**39**(4):336-341. DOI: 10.15537/smj.2018.4.21896

[24] MacDougall C. Aminoglycosides. In: Brunton LL, Hilal-Dandan R, Knollmann BC, editors. Goodman & Gilman's: The Pharmacological Basis of Therapeutics. 13th ed. New York, NY: McGraw-Hill Education; 2017

[25] Kotra LP, Haddad J, Mobashery S. Aminoglycosides: Perspectives on mechanisms of action and resistance and strategies to counter resistance. Antimicrobial Agents and Chemotherapy. 2000;**44**(12):3249-3256

[26] Busse HJ, Wostmann C, Barker EP. The bactericidal action of streptomycin: Membrane permeabilization caused by the insertion of mistranslated proteins into the cytoplasmic membrane of Escherichia coli and subsequent caging of the antibiotic inside the cells due to degradation of these proteins. Journal of General Microbiology. 1992;**138**(3):551-561. DOI: 10.1099/00221287-138-3-551

[27] Edson RS, Terrell CL. The aminoglycosides. Mayo Clinic Proceedings. 1999;**74**(5):519-528. DOI: 10.4065/74.5.519

[28] Scholar E. Streptomycin. xPharm Compr Pharmacol Ref2007. pp. 1-6. DOI: 10.1016/B978-008055232-3.62678-9

[29] Falagas M, Kasiakou S. Toxicity of polymyxins: A systematic review of the evidence from old and recent studies. Critical Care. 2006;**10**(1):R27. DOI: 10.1186/cc3995

[30] Zhou Y-F, Tao M-T, Feng Y, Yang R-S, Liao X-P, Liu Y-H, et al. Increased activity of colistin in combination with amikacin against Escherichia coli co-producing NDM-5 and MCR-1. The

Journal of Antimicrobial Chemotherapy. 2017;**72**(6):1723-1730. DOI: 10.1093/jac/dkx038

[31] Henderson JL, Polk RE, Kline BJ. In vitro inactivation of gentamicin, tobramycin, and netilmicin by carbenicillin, azlocillin, or mezlocillin. American Journal of Hospital Pharmacy. 1981;**38**(8):1167-1170

[32] Holt HA, Broughall JM, McCarthy M, Reeves DS. Interactions between aminoglycoside antibiotics and carbenicillin or ticarillin. Infection. 1976;**4**(2):107-109

[33] Tangy F, Moukkadem M, Vindimian E, Capmau M-L, Le Goffic F. Mechanism of action of gentamicin components characteristics of their binding to *Eschevichiu coli* ribosomes. European Journal of Biochemistry. 1985;**147**:381-386

[34] Leggett JE. Aminoglycosides. In: Mandell, Douglas, and Bennett's Principles and Practice of Infectious Diseases. 8th ed. US: Elsevier Health Bookshop; 2015. ISBN 9781455748013

[35] Pacifici GM. Clinical pharmacology of gentamicin in neonates: Regimen, toxicology and pharmacokinetics. MedicalExpress. 2015;**2**(5):1-9. DOI: 10.5935/MedicalExpress.2015.05.01

[36] Arup Laboratoties. Gentamicin, Random Level [Internet]. 2013. Available from: http://ltd.aruplab.com/tests/pub/0090130

[37] Medscape. Gentamicin Level: Reference Range, Collection and Panels, Background [Internet]. 2014. Available from: https://emedicine.medscape.com/article/2090086-overview

[38] Prayle A, Watson A, Fortnum H, Smyth A. Side effects of aminoglycosides on the kidney, ear and balance in cystic fibrosis. Thorax. 2010;**65**(7):654-658. DOI: 0.1136/thx.2009.131532

[39] Churchill DN, Seely J. Nephrotoxicity associated with combined gentamicin—Amphotericin B therapy. Nephron. 1977;**19**(3):176-181. DOI: 10.1159/000180883

[40] Mayordomo JI, Rivera F. Severe hypocalcaemia after treatment with oral clodronate and aminoglycoside. Annals of Oncology, the journal of the European Society for Medical Oncology. 1993;**4**(5):432-433

[41] Miller PD, Jamal SA, Evenepoel P, Eastell R, Boonen S. Renal safety in patients treated with bisphosphonates for osteoporosis: A review. Journal of Bone and Mineral Research. 2013;**28**(10):2049-2059. DOI: 10.1002/jbmr.2058

[42] Lawson DH, Tilstone WJ, Gray JM, Srivastava PK. Effect of furosemide on the pharmacokinetics of gentamicin in patients. Journal of Clinical Pharmacology. 1982;**22**(5-6):254-258

[43] Nakahama H, Fukuhara Y, Orita Y, Yamauchi A, Takama T, Kamada T. Furosemide accelerates gentamicin accumulation in cultured renal cells (LLC-PK1 cells). Nephron. 1989;**53**(2):138-141. DOI: 10.1159/000185726

[44] Gumbo T. Chemotherapy of tuberculosis, mycobacterium avium complex disease, and leprosy. In: Brunton LL, Hilal-Dandan R, Knollmann BC, editors. Goodman & Gilman's: The Pharmacological Basis of Therapeutics. 13th ed. New York, NY: McGraw-Hill Education; 2017

[45] Wilkins JJ, Savic RM, Karlsson MO, Langdon G, McIlleron H, Pillai G, et al. Population pharmacokinetics of rifampin in pulmonary tuberculosis patients, including a semimechanistic model to describe variable absorption. Antimicrobial Agents and Chemotherapy. 2008;**52**(6):2138-2148. DOI: 10.1128/AAC.00461-07

[46] Mahatthanatrakul W, Nontaput T, Ridtitid W, Wongnawa M, Sunbhanich M. Rifampin, a cytochrome P450 3A inducer, decreases plasma concentrations of antipsychotic risperidone in healthy volunteers. Journal of Clinical Pharmacy and Therapeutics. 2007;**32**(2):161-167. DOI: 10.1111/j.1365-2710.2007.00811.x

[47] Chawla PK, Udwadia ZF, Soman R, Mahashur AA, Amale RA, Dherai AJ, et al. Importance of therapeutic drug monitoring of rifampicin. The Journal of the Association of Physicians of India. 2016;**64**(8):68-72

[48] Martínez E, Collazos J, Mayo J. Hypersensitivity reactions to rifampin. Pathogenetic mechanisms, clinical manifestations, management strategies, and review of the anaphylactic-like reactions. Medicine. 1999;**78**(6):361-369

[49] Machado-Alba JE, Erazo-Bravo NJ, Gaviria-Mendoza A, Medina-Morales DA. Síndrome seudogripal en un paciente con terapia antituberculosa. Infection. 2016;**20**(3):176-179. DOI: 10.1016/j.infect.2015.11.002

[50] Verma AK, Singh A, Chandra A, Kumar S, Gupta RK. Rifampicin-induced thrombocytopenia. Indian Journal of Pharmacology. 2010;**42**(4):240-242. DOI: 10.4103/0253-7613.68432

[51] Chen J, Raymond K. Roles of rifampicin in drug-drug interactions: Underlying molecular mechanisms involving the nuclear pregnane X receptor. Annals of Clinical Microbiology and Antimicrobials. 2006;**5**:3. DOI: 10.1186/1476-0711-5-3

[52] Chang S-H, Chou I-J, Yeh Y-H, Chiou M-J, Wen M-S, Kuo C-T, et al. Association between use of non-vitamin K Oral anticoagulants with and without concurrent medications and risk of major bleeding in nonvalvular atrial fibrillation. Journal of the American Medical Association. 2017;**318**(13):1250. DOI: 10.1001/jama.2017.13883

[53] Park G, Bae SH, Park W-S, Han S, Park M-H, Shin S-H, et al. Drug-drug interaction of microdose and regular-dose omeprazole with a CYP2C19 inhibitor and inducer. Drug Design, Development and Therapy. 2017;**11**:1043-1053. DOI: 10.2147/DDDT.S131797

[54] Kim K-A, Park P-W, Liu K-H, Kim K-B, Lee H-J, Shin J-G, et al. Effect of rifampin, an inducer of CYP3A and P-glycoprotein, on the pharmacokinetics of risperidone. Journal of Clinical Pharmacology. 2008;**48**(1):66-72. DOI: 10.1177/0091270007309888

[55] Bolhuis MS, Panday PN, Pranger AD, Kosterink JGW, Alffenaar J-WC. Pharmacokinetic drug interactions of antimicrobial drugs: A systematic review on oxazolidinones, rifamycines, macrolides, fluoroquinolones, and beta-lactams. Pharmaceutics. 2011;**3**(4):865-913. DOI: 10.3390/pharmaceutics3040865

[56] MacDougall C. Sulfonamides, trimethoprim-sulfamethoxazole, quinolones, and agents for urinary tract infections. In: Brunton LL, Hilal-Dandan R, Knollmann BC, editors. Goodman & Gilman's: The Pharmacological Basis of Therapeutics. 13th ed. New York, NY: McGraw-Hill Education; 2017

[57] Drlica K, Zhao X. DNA gyrase, topoisomerase IV, and the 4-quinolones. Microbiology and Molecular Biology Reviews. 1997;**61**(3):377-392

[58] Etminan M, Brophy JM, Samii A. Oral fluoroquinolone use and risk of peripheral neuropathy: A pharmacoepidemiologic study. Neurology. 2014;**83**(14):1261-1263. DOI: 10.1212/WNL.0000000000000846

[59] Van der Linden PD, Sturkenboom MCJM, Herings RMC, Leufkens HMG, Rowlands S, Stricker BHC. Increased risk of achilles tendon rupture with quinolone antibacterial use, especially in elderly patients taking oral corticosteroids. Archives of Internal Medicine. 2003;**163**(15):1801-1807. DOI: 10.1001/archinte.163.15.1801

[60] Zabraniecki L, Negrier I, Vergne P, Arnaud M, Bonnet C, Bertin P, et al. Fluoroquinolone induced tendinopathy: Report of 6 cases. The Journal of Rheumatology. 1996;**23**(3):516-520

[61] Kang J, Wang L, Chen XL, Triggle DJ, Rampe D. Interactions of a series of fluoroquinolone antibacterial drugs with the human cardiac K+ channel HERG. Molecular Pharmacology. 2001;**59**(1):122-126

[62] Höffken G, Borner K, Glatzel PD, Koeppe P, Lode H. Reduced enteral absorption of ciprofloxacin in the presence of antacids. European Journal of Clinical Microbiology. 1985;**4**(3):345

[63] Shiba K, Sakai O, Shimada J, Okazaki O, Aoki H, Hakusui H. Effects of antacids, ferrous sulfate, and ranitidine on absorption of DR-3355 in humans. Antimicrobial Agents and Chemotherapy. 1992;**36**(10):2270-2274

[64] Prince RA, Casabar E, Adair CG, Wexler DB, Lettieri J, Kasik JE. Effect of quinolone antimicrobials on theophylline pharmacokinetics. Journal of Clinical Pharmacology. 1989;**29**(7):650-654. DOI: 10.1002/j.1552-4604.1989.tb03394.x

[65] Grasela TH, Dreis MW. An evaluation of the quinolone-theophylline interaction using the Food and Drug Administration spontaneous reporting system. Archives of Internal Medicine. 1992;**152**(3):617. DOI: 1001/archinte.1992.00400150127023

[66] Kalkut G. Sulfonamides and trimethoprim. Cancer Investigation. 1998;**16**(8):612-615

[67] Ho JM-W, Juurlink DN. Considerations when prescribing trimethoprim-sulfamethoxazole. Canadian Medical Association Journal. 2011;**183**(16):1851. DOI: 10.1503/CMAJ.111152

[68] Antoniou T, Gomes T, Mamdani MM, Juurlink DN. Trimethoprim/sulfamethoxazole-induced phenytoin toxicity in the elderly: A population-based study. British Journal of Clinical Pharmacology. 2011;**71**(4):544-549. DOI: 10.1111/j.1365-2125.2010.03866.x

[69] Schelleman H, Bilker W, Brensinger C, Han X, Kimmel S, Hennessy S. Warfarin with fluoroquinolones, sulfonamides, or azole antifungals: Interactions and the risk of hospitalization for gastrointestinal bleeding. Clinical Pharmacology and Therapeutics. 2008;**84**(5):581-588. DOI: 10.1038/clpt.2008.150

[70] Lane MA, Zeringue A, McDonald JR. Serious bleeding events due to warfarin and antibiotic co-prescription in a cohort of veterans. The American Journal of Medicine. 2014;**127**(7):657-663.e2. DOI: 10.1016/j.amjmed.2014.01.044

[71] Ahmed A, Stephens JC, Kaus CA, Fay WP. Impact of preemptive warfarin dose reduction on anticoagulation after initiation of trimethoprim-sulfamethoxazole or levofloxacin. Journal of Thrombosis and Thrombolysis. 2008;**26**(1):44-48. DOI: 10.1007/s11239-007-0164-z

[72] Dizbay M, Kilic S, Hizel K, Arman D. Tigecycline: Its potential for treatment of brucellosis. Scandinavian Journal of Infectious Diseases. 2007;**39**(5):432-434

[73] Solís García del Pozo J, Solera J. Systematic review and meta-analysis of randomized clinical trials in the treatment of human brucellosis. PLoS One. 2012;**7**(2):e32090

[74] Roushan MRH, Amiri MJS, Janmohammadi N, Hadad MS, Javanian M, Baiani M, et al. Comparison of the efficacy of gentamicin for 5 days plus doxycycline for 8 weeks versus streptomycin for 2 weeks plus doxycycline for 45 days in the treatment of human brucellosis: A randomized clinical trial. The Journal of Antimicrobial Chemotherapy. 2010;**65**(5):1028-1035

[75] Ranjbar M, Keramat F, Mamani M, Kia AR, Khalilian FO-S, Hashemi SH, et al. Comparison between doxycycline-rifampin-amikacin and doxycycline-rifampin regimens in the treatment of brucellosis. International Journal of Infectious Diseases. 2007;**11**(2):152-156

Chapter 6

Immunopathogenesis of Salmonellosis

Mashooq Ahmad Dar, Peerzada Tajamul Mumtaz, Shakil Ahmad Bhat, Qamar Taban, Shabir Ahmad Khan, Tufail Banday and Syed Mudasir Ahmad

Abstract

Salmonella is an intracellular pathogenic, gram-negative, facultative anaerobe and non-spore-forming and usually a motile bacillus that leads to salmonellosis in the host. It is a common food-borne disease that ranges from local gastrointestinal inflammation and diarrhoea to life-threatening typhoid fever and presents usually a serious threat to public health due to its socio-economic value. Inadequate sanitation and impure water help in the propagation of this disease. Despite advancement in the sanitation standards, *Salmonella* enters the food chain and affects communities globally. There is an immediate need to develop improved vaccines to minimise *Salmonella*-related illnesses. Some *Salmonella* serovars infect a wide range of hosts, while others are known to be host restricted. Many different factors determine the adaptability and host specificity of *Salmonella*. The host-pathogen interactions play a unique role in *Salmonella* invasion and progression which needs to be studied in detail. This chapter shall focus on our current understanding of *Salmonella* invasion, pathogenesis and interactions with the host, host specificity and adaptability.

Keywords: *Salmonella*, serovars, adaptability, specificity, invasion, non-typhoidal *Salmonella*, typhoidal *Salmonella*, immune response

1. Introduction

Salmonellae are facultative anaerobes and gram-negative, non-spore-forming and usually motile bacilli. Two species, namely, *Salmonella enterica and Salmonella bongori*, belong to genus *Salmonella*. *Salmonella enterica* is further subdivided into six subspecies that are distinguished by variations in O (somatic) and H (flagellar) antigens with at least 2500 serotypes. *S. enterica* subsp. *enterica* comprises of more than half of the known serotypes [1]. New serotypes are being discovered increasing the serotype complexity. Approximately 99% of the *Salmonella* serotypes that infect humans and other mammals belong to *S. enterica* subspecies. These serovars are mostly the inhabitants of intestinal tract of humans and other organisms that include reptiles, birds and insects. At farm level, sources of bacterial contamination are faecal matter, litter, feed and soil [2]. *Salmonella* most commonly causes food-borne illnesses worldwide; the two commonly associated foods are eggs and poultry meat [3]. Serovars *S.* Enteritidis, *S.* Typhimurium, *S.* Heidelberg and *S.* Newport are linked to such food-borne diseases, with farm animals being reservoirs for these serotypes [4, 5]. Salmonellosis is a big socio-economic threat worldwide that causes considerable mortality and morbidity in both humans and animals [6]. Most of the human-related diseases are food-borne, and exposure to these bacteria at different places has also been linked to human salmonellosis. The most orthodox mode of bacterial transmission is the faecal-oral route. Once the bacteria are transmitted, the initial site for bacterial infection is the small intestine. Following infection, different manifestations that arise range from gastroenteritis to enteric fever [7].

2. Epidemiology

The extensive investigation of the associated epidemiological risk factors that make an organism a persistent *Salmonella* carrier needs to be carried out. Non-typhoidal *Salmonella* (NTS) infections that cause self-limiting manifestations are the most common to occur globally. In comparison, typhoidal *Salmonella* (TS) causing enteric fever leads to a high rate of mortality and morbidity that predominantly affects the underdeveloped countries [8]. Recent studies conclude that *Salmonella* Paratyphi A incidences have risen especially in South East Asia where approximately half of the TS-infected enteric fever patients are reported to be infected with *S.* Paratyphi A [9]. The food chain can get contaminated at any stage, and most of the transmission can occur by contaminated foods like poultry and dairy-related products. Apart from contaminated food products, NTS transmission can also result from person-to-person contact or from contact with other bacterial reservoirs. After gaining entry into the host, both TS and NTS serovars initially invade the intestinal epithelium of the small intestine.

3. Diseases caused by *Salmonella* infection

Salmonella species cause a varying number of clinical manifestations in the host that can range from self-limiting gastroenteritis typically associated with non-typhoidal *Salmonella* (NTS) to typhoidal or paratyphoidal fevers, which can be life-threatening [6].

3.1 Typhoidal *Salmonella* (TS)

Humans are exclusive hosts for serovars such as *S.* Typhi, *S.* Sendai and *S.* Paratyphi A, B and C. These serovars are known as typhoidal serovars (TS) that can cause enteric fever/typhoidal/paratyphoidal fevers. Enteric fever is a systemic disease that is highly invasive and life threatening and is endemic in the developing world. Within an incubation period of around 2 weeks, bacteraemia occurs, which is marked by fever and malaise. The symptoms that start to appear after a week include fever, malaise, nausea, dry cough and abdominal discomfort. Common symptoms include tender abdomen, coated tongue, splenomegaly and hepatomegaly [10]. As the lack of adequate water and sanitation facilities in the developing countries help in the spread of *Salmonella* through faecal-oral route [11], so to prevent typhoidal *Salmonella* transmission, societal standards need to be improved. The development of improved societal infrastructures is generally cost prohibitive in developing countries, hence, having little significance in reducing the disease frequency. In comparison, the development of effective and safe typhoidal vaccines can have a significant effect on reducing typhoidal cases.

3.2 Non-typhoidal *Salmonella* (NTS)

Many industrialised and underdeveloped countries across the globe face a significant threat of non-typhoidal *Salmonella* (NTS). Worldwide, about 93.8 million gastroenteritis cases arise from *Salmonella* infections leading to 1.5 million deaths annually [7]. In infants, young, aged and immunologically compromised subjects NTS cause invasive bacterial infection [12, 13]. After post infection with NTS, symptoms that arise last for about 10 days that triggers a massive inflammatory response involving the release of pro-inflammatory cytokines and chemokines. The human NTS patients have higher serum levels of different interleukins and cytokines like IL-18, IL-12, IL-10, IL-15, TNF- α and IFN γ [14]. Non-typhoidal *Salmonella* serovars can cause severe extra-intestinal disease in patients with deficiencies in type 1 cytokine pathways such as IFN-γ/IL-12/IL-23 especially IL-12 abnormalities. Effective vaccination against NTS is lacking as there is a greater variance among different serovars. So, for generating effective vaccines against NTS, knowledge regarding different target antigens needs to be studied in detail. To disrupt the bacterial transmission and the incidence, effective preventive measures such as improving sanitation, hygiene and drinking clean water must be taken into consideration. Different host specificities and adaptability are shown by different *Salmonella* serovars that shall be discussed in detail.

4. Host specificity and adaptation

Salmonellosis susceptibly ranges from organism to organism and can occur in almost all animal species, but the clinical severity of this disease varies among the hosts. There are only specific serovars that cause severe clinical manifestations in their specific hosts [15]. Although most of the serovars of *S. enterica* subspecies cause infections which give rise to gastroenteritis that lasts for short durations, some serovars lead to severe systemic illness in humans and animals accompanied by septicaemia, fever and in some cases abortion. Based on the host specificity, these serovars can be grouped into two categories: the first category consists of serovars that are single-host restricted and the second category infecting a broad range of hosts. Different factors can be considered for grouping different serovars under the above-mentioned categories. Also, serovar pathogenicity and host epidemiology define host specificity. Keeping the above factors into account, different serovars have been grouped into three major groups. The first group comprises of serovars that mainly infect cattle and pigs but can also infect other animals including humans in some accidental cases. In this group, *S. choleraesuis* and dublin have been included that cause systemic diseases in the above-mentioned hosts. In humans and other animals, clinical symptoms may not be visible, thus making them asymptomatic. *Salmonella* carriers that can shed the bacteria in the surroundings thus leading to increased risk for susceptible hosts are also known as host-adapted serovars (HA) [16]. The second group infects specific hosts and is collectively known as host-restricted (HR) serovars. The HR serovars cause systemic diseases and can sometimes prove lethal in their hosts that include poultry, humans, sheep, equine and pigs. This group includes *S. gallinarum*, *S.* typhi, *S.* abortus and *S.* abortusequi. They interfere with the environment of their hosts in a way that paves their way for invading the host. This ability to cause mammalian abortions and loss in poultry egg production is due to their remarkable ability to multiply in the foetal tissues [16–18]. The serovars of the third group are known as unrestricted serovars that are of zoonotic, epidemiological importance and impose a great threat to many animals and humans. The serovars of this group that are of much clinical importance are *S. typhimurium* and *S. enteritidis* [18]. These cause mild symptoms in the adult host, and sometimes the host does not show any visible clinical symptoms despite infection. They severely invade young hosts as compared to adult hosts because the adult hosts have a well-built immune system that hinders the invasion by these serovars [16]. The host specificity and adaptability of different serovars are a complex process and involve many molecular mechanisms. The exact mechanisms are poorly studied, but certain factors have been found to be responsible for determining host specificity and adaptability.

4.1 Factors determining *Salmonella* host specificity and adaptation

Although the exact mechanisms to host specificity have not been fully deciphered, the existing evidence shows that serovars act independently of each other at the various phases of infection. The expression of serovar's pathogenicity is affected by the environmental and genetic factors influencing each host during adaptation [19]. Each HA/HR serovar must overcome the encountered specific and nonspecific immune mechanisms. Thus, pathogenicity of HA serovars results from the development of ways helping their survival in a host. Examples of this are serovars of *S. enterica* subsp. *enterica*, which have developed the ability to evade the immune mechanisms of warm-blooded animals. They have, during their evolution, acquired the ability to modify to their favour the physiological functions of their host, such as intracellular engulfment, apoptosis, transfer of antigens by M (microfold) cells, migration of macrophages and lymphocytes in the reticuloendothelial system and others [20]. A well-known serovar *S. typhi* has evolved to survive in human macrophages making it pathogenic to man, but not to mice [21]. Serovars such as the HR *S. typhi*, *S. gallinarum* and *S. abortusovis* show high tropism for the lymphatic organs of their hosts, thereby regulating their natural host's biological environment in their favour [19]. By anchoring to the cells of the bone marrow, PPs and bursa of Fabricius in the development of B cells, thus immune response is affected. The result of such interactions, particularly in adult animals, helps in the establishment of chronic or subclinical infection and thus prolonged subclinical excretion, but they do not help in the development of severe gastroenteritis [22]. Serovars not fully adapted to evade the mature immune system lack specificity, causing deadly systemic disease in adult animals by invading their defence mechanisms compared to HR serovars [20]. HR serovars are mildly enteropathogenic compared to the unrestricted serovars; thus, they do not cause intestinal inflammation [23]. It has also been shown that the ability of a serovar to metabolise a wide range of amino acids adds to its virulence and is thought to be closely related [24, 25]; however, HR or HA serovars have most likely evolved independently. On the other hand, the heterogenicity of serovars in relation to different metabolic profiles facilitates either the completion of the pathway to infection [26] or, when lacking specificity, it is favouring host adaptation [19]. The process of *Salmonella* host adaptation is believed to be involving either the loss of genes or the acquisition of novel genetic elements that encode specific virulence factors, and thus an inconvenience is observed frequently in the pathogenic strains. Best examples of host specificity dependent on gene deletions are, perhaps, of *S. enteritidis*, Typhimurium, Choleraesuis, Gallinarum, Abortusovis, Pullorum and Paratyphi C [27]. Genome sequencing of HA/HR serovars, such as Typhi, Gallinarum, Choleraesuis and the newly emerging in sub-Saharan Africa invasive strains of *S.* Typhi, has divulged that these have encountered extensive gene deletions and truncation [28, 29]. In systemically noninvasive *Salmonella*, the majority of lost genes have functional orthologues, which play a key role in intestinal colonisation, thus resulting in the loss of an intestinal multiplication cycle for narrowly host-adapted *Salmonellae* followed by a concurrent acquisition of mechanisms helping the microorganism to survive in a systemic niche [30]. Point mutations, horizontal gene transfer, positive selection and genome degradation could be responsible for a differential pathoadaptive evolution of some *Salmonella* serovars [31]. It appears from the analysis of the mannose-sensitive fimbrial adhesin FimH that even single amino acid replacement, resulting in specific structural mutations in FimH variants of HA serovars, plays an important role in the differential adaptive evolution of *Salmonella* spp. Thus, activation or inactivation of mannose-specific adhesive properties in different systemically invasive serovars reflects the dynamic trajectories of adaptation to the biological environment of a specific host. Furthermore, phylogenetic analysis has indicated that these mutations are, most likely, of a convergent nature (common pathogenic traits incorporated into different genetic backgrounds) and occur under strong positive selection, illustrative of the role of point amino acid changes for HA *Salmonella*. Certainly, deep study for the molecular composition of flagella, chemotaxis genes [32], fimbriae and bacteriophages and the presence of virulence plasmids and subtypes of each specific serovar is needed, to understand mechanisms of pathogenicity and host specificity [19]. Correlation between some phage types of *S.* Typhi with their hosts has shown considerable host specificity [33]. However, the majority of phage types studied had a broad host range, perhaps, suggesting a phage transfer of virulent genes between hosts, leading eventually to host specificity. The unrestricted serovar Typhimurium may comprise a spectrum of variants differing in regard to virulence, reflecting a summation of the spatial and/or temporal selective pressures within a particular host [34]. *Salmonella* Typhimurium strains derived from animal cases were also virulent in mice, whereas many strains derived from a clinically ill man lacked this ability. Of interest was that many derived from human gastroenteritis lacked the *Salmonella* virulence plasmid, present in all animal strains and strains isolated from human bacteraemia. Furthermore, some strains harbouring the virulence plasmid isolated from the man were avirulent in mice, and the opposite was observed with those derived from animals. Altogether, isolates of a specific bacterial serovar obtained from human salmonellosis are different from those isolated from animals. This means that selective pressure within a specific host gives rise to bacterial strain variants that exhibit different pathogenicity determinants, thus varying degree of pathogenicity. Similarly, serovars of *S. enterica* subsp. *enterica*, associated with disease in mammals and birds, show different degrees of adaptability. Pathogenicity determinants, such as the FimH adhesins, play an important role. Type 1 FimH adhesins are expressed by serovars of *S. enterica* isolated from mammalian and avian hosts, while type 2 FimH is expressed exclusively by the avian-adapted serovar Gallinarum. Allelic variation of the *S. enterica* FimH adhesin directs host-cell-specific recognition, thus selectively binding to mammalian or avian receptors [35]. The distribution of SPIs, fimbriae operons and virulence plasmids has shown that various combinations of virulent determinants formed during the evolution of the microorganism are needed for a variant to become pathogenic in a particular range of host species. Mutations horizontally transmitted could have helped the development of host specificity by helping *Salmonella* serovars to harbour unique virulence factors [36]. Molecular and phylogenetic analyses of the SPI genes showed that these encode for translocon proteins (SipD, SseC and SseD) present on both *Salmonella* pathogenicity islands SPI-1 and SPI-2 and also encode an effector protein that inhibits the MAPK pathway of the host cells [37]. In addition, they encode effector proteins (SseF and SifA) important in placing the *Salmonella*-containing vacuole (SCV) in a juxtanuclear position. The products of SPI genes interact directly with the host and modulate its functions, thus favouring host specificity. Another study of the SPI genes has shown the close evolutionary relatedness between serovars Gallinarum and Enteritidis [38], although the former is highly adapted (restricted) to poultry and is the only known non-motile serovar, while serovar Enteritidis is unrestricted. Analysis of the functions of genes associated to SPI-1 showed that virulence genes might have evolved under positive selection imposed by a serovar's respective host(s) contributing to the different host specificity observed between different serovars. This has displayed that a close similarity of core regions exists within as well as among different serovar genomes [39]. In particular, genomic comparisons of HR and HA serovars show that genomic degradation is a common evolutionary mechanism for host adaptation and increased pathogenicity [39, 40]. Others have shown that host restriction and change of ecological niche are associated with the accumulation of pseudogenes and an overall reduction in genome size [28]. For example, *S.* Typhi and Paratyphi A are restricted to the man and cause a similar systemic disease. Genome sequence similarity between Typhi and Paratyphi A serovars and their different pathogenicity when compared to the unrestricted serovars of *S. enterica* have been attributed to a relatively recent recombination of a quarter of their genomes, making the aggregation of pseudogenes a key feature of convergent evolution for these and other HA pathogens [31]. Another example supporting the role of convergent evolution is serovar Paratyphi C, which has diverged from the same ancestor as serovar Choleraesuis, by accumulating genomic novelty during its adaptation process to man. The genomic analysis of these two *Salmonella* serovars has revealed a highly similar genomic construction between the two and their distinct pathogenic features, making them excellent models for studying *Salmonella's* host adaptation and pathogenic divergence [39]. Hence, *Salmonella* adaptation to a particular host species is a complex phenomenon, which depends, apparently, on a large number of gene products. The prowess of understanding host-pathogen interactions requires analysis of the physiological associations between various animal species and genetic composition.

5. *Salmonella* invasion

After ingestion of *Salmonella* by the host organism, it travels from the stomach and invades intestinal epithelial cells. Bacterial recognition generates an inflammatory response following the recruitment of a variety of bone-marrow-derived phagocytes [41]. The ability of *Salmonella* to access intestinal epithelium (M cells) is due to the presence of virulence genes encoded by *Salmonella* pathogenicity island 1 (SPI-1). Proteins that are encoded by SPI-1 form a needle-like Type III secretion system which allows the transport of several bacterial proteins into the host cell cytosol. These proteins induce changes in the host cells such as the rearrangement of the cytoskeleton and cell membrane and disconnection of epithelial cell junctions, facilitating bacterial invasion [42]. The primary site of *Salmonella* infection occurs at specialised microfold, or M cells, that are dispersed among the enterocytes, covering the follicle-associated epithelium (FAE) of the Peyer's patch (PP) [43] (**Figure 1**). *Salmonella* is considered to preferentially invade PPs in the distal ileum, but in practice, all intestinal PPs will harbour bacteria after moderate-to-high-dose infection. Once *Salmonella* is penetrated, it initiates destruction of M cell which disrupts the mucosal barrier and allows additional entry of bacteria through neighbouring enterocytes [43]. This process is extremely efficient, with M-cell penetration followed by M-cell destruction. Once access to PP via FAE is gained, invading bacteria enter the lymphatic system where they interact with professional killing cells (phagocytes) that ultimately determine the fate of the infection. Phagocytes are involved in both oxygen-dependent and oxygen-independent killing of the engulfed bacteria. During intestinal NTS infection, the release of reactive oxygen

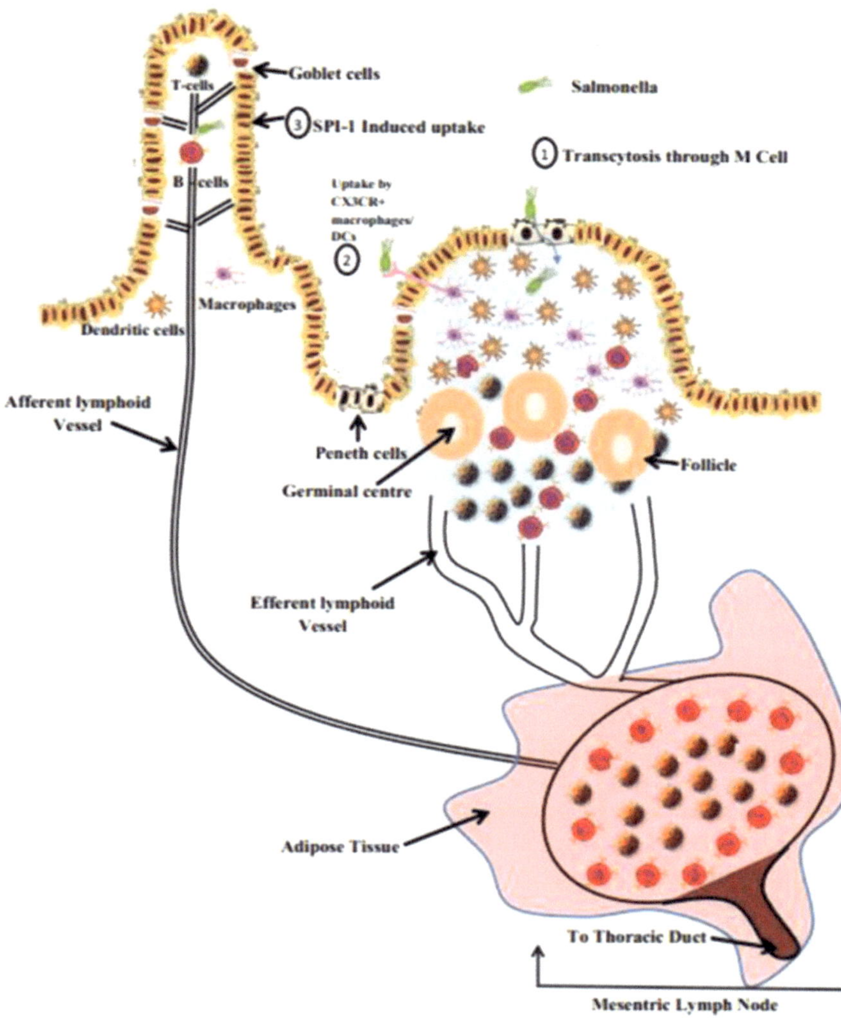

Figure 1.
Salmonella entry in intestinal epithelial cells. SPI-1 facilitates uptake and destruction of M cells, SILTs. After invasion of under tissues, Salmonella is taken by phagocytes and transported to mesenteric lymph nodes.

and nitrogen species creates a highly oxidative environment which is not permissive for the growth of bacteria. The subepithelial dome also contains dendritic cell (DC) subsets apart from macrophage populations, each of which can phagocytise the bacteria and then undergo apoptosis through a caspase-1-dependent mechanism [44]. Consequently, during *Salmonella* infection, the number of obligate anaerobes decline in the gut. Also, host-signalling environment is highly crucial for the disease development initiated by contact between microbe and host cells in various tissues, largely mediated by cytokine signalling. These cytokines aid in initiating and regulating the innate and adaptive branches of the immune response against *Salmonella*. In order to avoid damage to the host, the release of pro- and anti-inflammatory cytokines must be balanced [45]. M cells are not only abundant in PPs; they also predominate in other intestinal locations and so can, therefore, mediate infection of non-PP intestinal tissues (**Figure 1**). The most likely non-PP entry route is through the bacterial invasion of solitary intestinal lymphoid tissues (SILTs), which are heterogeneous intestinal lymphoid aggregates found in mice and humans that contain certain features of PPs, including the presence of FAE-containing M cells [46, 47]. These SILTs are invaded by bacteria in a much similar manner as described above for PPs [48]. SILTs can be important in humans since in a study of typhoid patients, both PPs and SILTs showed inflammation. It has also been reported that intravillous M cells, which are sparsely located along the intestinal tract, may serve as a portal of entry for invasive *Salmonella* bacteria [49, 50] (**Figure 1**).

5.1 Alternative route for invasion

The main entry route described above involve, bacterial interactions with M cells, the possibility is that it can invade the host by an alternative route that does not involve M cells. A population of phagocytes in the lamina propria capture bacteria directly from luminal contents which also allow bacterial entry [51, 52]. This is for those bacteria that lack SPI-1 genes as this route does not involve M cell-mediated uptake. These cells might have been referred to as DCs, but as this is not clear [53, 54], they will be referred to as lamina propria phagocytes in this chapter. Although this pathway has now become an alternative to our general understanding of bacterial entry through M cells, the physiological importance of this route to systemic salmonellosis is poorly defined. The compelling evidence for a non-M-cell pathway is largely derived from microbiological and immunological investigations. Recent interest was stimulated by demonstrating that strains lacking SPI-1 and the fimbrial lpfC gene that did not normally infect mice retained the ability to infect mice in a CD18-dependent manner and were rapidly detected in the blood after oral inoculation [55, 56]. This extremely rapid dissemination to the blood and lack of serovar specificity might be due to bacterial entry in the bloodstream of the host through abrasions caused during gavage. Many cervical lymph node infection cases that attributed to the entry through mucosal abrasions during gavage were revealed through bacterial imaging system [57]. Expression of the SPI-2 type-III secretion system effector protein (SrfH) of bacteria was required for very early dissemination of bacteria to the blood and spleen [58]. This finding supports the idea that rapid entry through an alternative pathway involves active processes, so, therefore, it is important to examine this route from a microbiological perspective. In vitro studies demonstrated that DCs could capture bacteria by extending processes between the tight junctions of a monolayer and the apical surface of epithelial cells [59]. Subsequently, a similar process was directly visualised in vivo when CX3CR1-expressing phagocytes were detected extending transepithelial dendrites in the lamina propria, and the number of dendrites increased in the terminal ileum after infection [60]. So, these studies suggested an alternative entry model, whereby *Salmonella* might commonly access the intestinal lamina propria by cell sampling, as large numbers of bacteria were detected within the lamina propria [60]. However, *Salmonella* is not normally recoverable in large numbers from the lamina propria unless the bacterial flora is first depleted before infection [48]. Also, the formation of transepithelial dendrites is dispensable for the uptake of other pathogenic microorganisms [61]. More importantly, it has been demonstrated that CX3CR1+ lamina propria cells are unlikely to migrate to the mesenteric lymph nodes (MLN) and have poor immunostimulatory capacity [53]. Thus, CX3CR1+ cells most likely represent a population of non-migrating phagocytes that provide innate immune defence against infection within the lamina propria. Surprisingly, the role of cell-mediated uptake has not been examined carefully in PPs or in SILTs, but still, phagocytic cells are often found in association with the epithelium of tissues [48, 62]. In summary, a prominent role for M cell-mediated intestinal entry by *Salmonella* is played both in the PPs and SILTs, whereas *Salmonella* entry of the lamina propria and the mechanisms like immune activation and bacterial dissemination associated with this pathway of entry remain largely speculative.

6. *Salmonella* infection of mesenteric lymph nodes (MLNs) and systemic tissues

After initial invasion through PPs, the ultimate fate of infection is decided in the lymphatic system. The indication for the bacterial migration is based on our understanding of the lymph and the conjectural finding that bacteria are detected initially in PPs, followed by the MLN and finally the liver and spleen [63, 64]. *Salmonella* after getting access to efferent lymphatics reaches the systemic tissues via the thoracic duct and blood after reaching the MLN [65, 66]. The immune cell population that aids in the transport of bacteria to the blood and other tissues is not well known; however, intestinal DCs are usually considered as a possibility. The majority of bacteria were found free in the lymph or were associated with non-DC phagocytes [67], but it is not clear whether this also occurs during exit from the MLN. Disseminated bacteria show a tropism of tissues that contain a high number of phagocytic cells, and in most circumstances, this involves the spleen, liver, and bone marrow [65, 68]. Disruption of erythropoiesis and splenomegaly by *Salmonella* can be explained majorly by the expansion of immature erythrocytes in the spleen in an erythropoietin-dependent manner. Cancer studies have demonstrated that bacteria preferentially accumulate in primary and metastatic tumours [69, 70], suggesting that it does not have a precise organ tropism but finds tissues that contain a sufficient number of cells that support bacterial replication. The large size of the spleen, liver, and bone marrow means that these tissues gradually comprise the major sites of bacterial replication [71, 72]. Thus, *Salmonella* causes systemic infection that uses intestinal lymphoid tissues as a portal of entry. Also that bacteria clearance from the host and resistance to secondary infection requires the coordinated action of both systemic and mucosal immunity.

7. Host innate immune response to *Salmonella*

After phagocytosis by macrophages, *Salmonella* can survive and replicate within modified intracellular vesicles, termed as *Salmonella*-containing vacuoles (SCV) [73, 74]. The ability of *Salmonella* to survive within the phagosome is mediated by SPI-2, which prevents movement of RNS and ROS into the phagosome where the bacteria reside [75, 76]. In addition, *Salmonella* phoP/phoQ regulon inhibits fusion of the SCV with toxic lysosomes and endosomes [77]. The natural resistance-associated macrophage protein encoding gene, which enables macrophages to transport ions into the SCV, provides resistance/susceptibility to infection [78]. Survival of bacteria intracellularly within tissue phagocytes is a prerequisite to the bacterial virulence, and bacterial mutants that cannot survive and replicate within macrophages are attenuated for virulence [79]. The initial invasion induces a massive inflammatory response, characterised by recruitment of neutrophils, DCs, inflammatory monocytes and macrophages [48, 80]. Neutrophils follow the chemokine gradient to the gut and extravagate into the mucosa. As they encounter and eliminate the bacteria by mechanisms that are not yet fully elucidated [81], neutrophils are believed to be important in preventing dissemination of the bacteria from the intestine to systemic tissues, so the patients with low neutrophil levels have a high risk of bacteraemia during infection with NTS strains [82]. Also, that depletion of neutrophils allows extracellular growth of bacteria, suggesting that neutrophils confine and reduce bacterial replication immediately after entry. Inflammatory monocytes are an important source of antimicrobial factors, such as TNFs and inducible NO synthase, during the initial stages of infection [80]. Myd88-dependent chemokine production within the PPs drives the recruitment of these inflammatory cells [81]. Indeed, *Salmonella* expresses several pathogen-associated molecular patterns (PAMPs), including lipopolysaccharide (LPS) and flagellin, which can be detected by Toll-like receptors (TLRs) expressed by enterocytes and phagocytes [83]. Also, macrophages after sensing cytosolic flagellin through NLRC4 (also known as Ipaf) activate caspase-1 and induce the production of IL-18 (pro-inflammatory) [84, 85]. Dendritic cells are professional antigen-presenting cells and increase the expression of MHC class II and the co-stimulatory molecules CD86, CD80 and CD40 by responding to the recognition of *Salmonella* LPS or flagellin [86, 87]. DCs present antigen to naive $CD4^+$ T cells, thus providing a vital link between innate immune responses and the induction of adaptive immunity. In the PPs, flagellin also induces the secretion of the inflammatory chemokine CCL20, which is an important ligand for CCR6 [88]. This response activates an early process whereby CCR6-expressing DCs are recruited to the FAE, for efficient activation of $CD4^+$ T cells [89].

8. Host-adaptive immune response to *Salmonella*

Adaptive immune response to *Salmonella* can be mediated via early $CD4^+$ T-cell activation. Due to the small size of intestinal lymphoid tissues and low frequency of naive $CD4^+$ T cells specific for any given antigen [90], detecting initial bacterial specific T-cell activation in these tissues is challenging. However, studies with T-cell receptor transgenic mice visualised the processes of bacterial specific $CD4^+$ T cells responding to oral infection [64, 91]. An artificially elevated naive precursor frequency of $CD4^+$ T cells at a high dose of infection provides the most accurate assessment of *Salmonella*-specific $CD4^+$ T-cell activation [92]. The earliest *Salmonella*-specific $CD4^+$ T-cell activation occurs within the MLN after oral infection but usually peaks few hours after that in the PPs [91]. At very early time points, $CD4^+$ T cells were not found to be activated in any other secondary lymphoid tissues [89], suggesting that whatever the explanation for early bacterial dissemination to blood as discussed above, no early adaptive immune response is initiated outside the gut-associated lymphoid tissue. Interestingly, the T-cell receptor transgenic model used recognises a bacterial peptide from the carboxy-terminal region of flagellin [93] which is also a ligand for TLR5 [94]. Generally, the early activation of flagellin-specific $CD4^+$ T cells in the PPs is representative of the naive $CD4^+$ response to other bacterial antigens [95, 96]. However, this is difficult to demonstrate conclusively as very few, naturally occurring bacterial specific MHC class-II peptides are known [97]. Interestingly, activation of $CD4^+$ T cells in the MLN is also dependent on $CD11c^+$ DCs and CCR6, indicating that T-cell activation in the MLN and PP has similar requirements. The evidence clearly suggests that the MLNs are an important site for immune protection during the course of *Salmonella* infection. Indeed, after MLNs were surgically removed, there was an elevated bacterial load and severe immunopathology in the liver [98]. The importance was also highlighted using a relapsing model of murine typhoid in which primary infection returns after apparent antibiotic clearance [57]. Although MLN is often considered a potential site of bacterial accumulation [99, 100], it acts as a protective firewall, preventing bacterial dissemination and relapsing *Salmonella* infection.

9. Host effector responses against *Salmonella*

The development of robust protective immunity against *Salmonella* infection requires the coordination of B and T cells. One hundred and sixteen $CD4^+$ T cells have a critical role in clearing the primary infection and are also required for acquired resistance to secondary infection [100]. In contrast, B cells are dispensable for resolving primary infection but are required for protection against secondary challenge [101]. There is a massive expansion of *Salmonella*-specific CD4⁺ T cells and rapid acquisition of Th1 effector functions, i.e. the enhanced ability to secrete INF-γ, TNF α and IL-2 upon restimulation [102] (**Figure 2**). These activated Th1 cells can be clearly detected a week after infection, which is consistent with the rapid tempo of $CD4^+$ T-cell activation. Optimal expansion of Th1 cells have been shown to require expression of both programmed death ligand-1 (PD-L1) and the TNF receptor family members, OX40 and CD30. Appropriately, expansion of activated Th1 cells eventually comprises ~50% of all $CD4^+$ T cells few weeks after infection [103]. Furthermore, Th1 cells are capable of responding to innate signals such as *Salmonella* LPS by secreting cytokines [104]. This innate response is unexpected as effector Th1 cells are normally stimulated only after recognition of cognate peptide and MHCs [105]. This innate immune responsiveness suggests a means by which the host can rapidly produce INF-γ to activate macrophages within an infected tissue, even if bacteria are capable of inhibiting antigen presentation by infected phagocytes [106]. Despite the rapid and efficient development of Th1 effector cells, there is actually little evidence that suggests their contribution to bacterial clearance during primary infection. Thus, it was found that when $CD4^+$ or $CD4^+$ Th1 cells were completely absent, bacterial growth enhanced a few weeks after infection which indicates that Th1 cells contribute little to regulate bacterial growth before this point [107]. Many in vitro studies point to an inhibitory effect of *Salmonella* on antigen presentation to naive T cells in vitro [108], but in vivo, there is no effect on *Salmonella*-specific $CD4^+$ expansion [109]. In contrast, the gradual loss of effector $CD4^+$ T cells detected in the process of *Salmonella* infection that required the presence of live bacteria and the expression of SPI-2 genes indicated that the effector function of cells is specifically

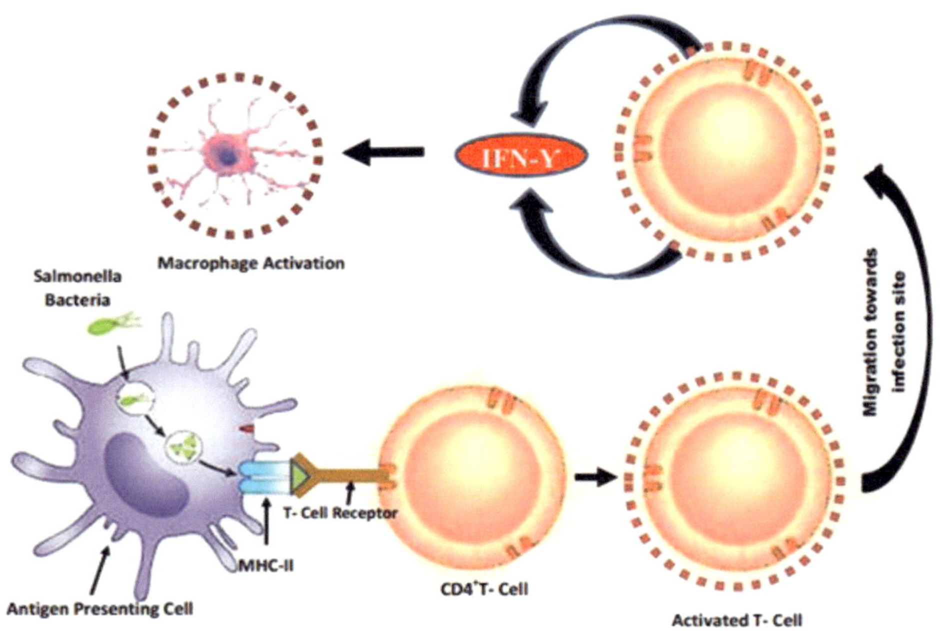

Figure 2.
Induction of IFN γ production by Salmonella-specific $CD4^+$T cells. Expansion of activated $CD4^+$T cells in secondary lymphoid tissues which in turn produces IFNγ at infection sites. Production of IFNγ finally activates macrophages.

inhibited by actively replicating bacteria [110]. Effector Th1 cells are effective in providing immunity to salmonellosis [111]; however, effector CD4⁺ subsets including regulatory T cells (Tregs) and Th17 cells are also known to contribute. Tregs arise from the thymus or develop after naive T-cell activation in the presence of TNF β which suppresses effector T-cell responses [112]. In contrast, Th17 cells arise from naive CD4⁺ T-cell stimulation in the presence of IL-6 and TNF-β and are important in mediating immunity against extracellular bacterial infections [113, 114]. During the development of Th1 cells and Tregs after infection, it was found that changes in the cogency of Tregs reduced the efficacy of Th1 responses and increased bacterial growth [102]. After oral infection with *Salmonella*, cytokines associated with Th17 cells, IL-17 and IL-22 are rapidly produced within the intestinal mucosa [115], and the production is induced by innate responses to infection rather than Th17 cells, however, still indicating the potential for Th17 cytokines to participate in intestinal defence against bacteria. In vivo, production of IL-22 dependent on IL12B, rather than IL-17, contributed to bacterial clearance [116]. Taken together, it is suggested that Th17 cells contribute additionally to protection against *Salmonella* infection by not only initiating or enhancing neutrophil infiltration to intestinal tissues but by the production of antimicrobial peptides by the epithelium which is effective against luminal bacteria as well [117]. In summary, it has been suggested that Th17 cells have an additional role in defence against *Salmonella* in the intestine and a role for Tregs in modulating the potency of *Salmonella*-specific Th1 cells in vivo.

10. Host antibody (Ab) response against *Salmonella*

Salmonella-specific B-cell responses contribute to bacterial clearance in the hosts [39, 120, 121]. Although the bacteria are generally found within SCV in phagocytic cells, there is a short period during the infection cycle when bacteria are expected to be extracellular. *Salmonella* is not only tightly associated with mononuclear phagocytes in vivo [118] but also induces these infected cells to undergo apoptosis [44]. After cell death, bacteria are presumably found in the extracellular compartment before infecting a neighbouring phagocyte. Thus, antibody might have direct access to the bacteria during this short period of time and prevent cell-to-cell transmission [92]. Bacterial colonisation obstructs the bacterial opsonization with *Salmonella*-specific Ab [119]. The Ab also plays a role in amplifying the processing and presentation of antigens to CD4⁺ T cells, thus affecting the Th1 response [120]. B-cell innate immune response to TLR-specific ligands is necessary for the development of Th1 responses in vivo [121]. New findings also suggest the suppression of protective immunity through B-cell MyD88 pathway during infection [122]. Therefore, innate immune signalling in B cells contributes to an important regulatory function but requires further analysis. The presence of *Salmonella*-specific Ab IgA in the intestinal mucosa may also prevent or reduce bacterial penetration of the intestinal barrier [123]. However, which of these mechanisms makes the greatest contribution to protective immunity is yet to be deciphered, but an important role for Ab is also suggested from human studies [124]. Although the specificity of Ab responses is undefined, Abs specific for the LPS O-antigen, flagellin, Vi capsular polysaccharide (ViCPS) antigen and outer membrane porin protein (OmpD) are all believed to be protective [125].

11. Conclusion

Members belonging to genus *Salmonella* are the major intestinal pathogens of human beings and animals. The increased food production and growth in human populations have led to the increase in dissemination potential of these ubiquitous microorganisms. Due to the systemic nature of some infections, where many tissues get involved to display immunity to specific infection, salmonellosis and the immune response that results are pliable. Deciphering the pathogenesis of invasive salmonellosis may hopefully lead to potential therapeutic treatment strategies that are urgently required in light of propagating antimicrobial resistance. Future studies must focus on the identification of molecular targets of *Salmonella* virulence factors during intracellular life in immune cells and designate the molecular mechanisms of interference. This would impart a novel perception into the cell biology of DCs and other immune cells. Furthermore, understanding the intracellular life of *Salmonella* may lead to new advancement in generating reliable vaccines against infections, to wield *Salmonella* strains as live carriers for recombinant vaccines and to evolve novel forms of treatment that target the function of specific virulence factors. Further explorations to clarify the contribution of genes differently represented/expressed in the genomes of various *Salmonella* serotypes during infection are required.

Abbreviations

NTS	non-typhoidal *Salmonella*
TS	typhoidal *Salmonella*
HA	host-adapted serovars
HR	host restricted
FAE	follicle-associated epithelium
PP	Peyer's patch
DC	dendritic cells
MHC	major histocompatibility complex
SPI	*Salmonella* pathogenicity island
SCV	*Salmonella*-containing vacuoles
MLN	mesenteric lymph nodes
PAMPs	pathogen-associated molecular patterns
LPS	lipopolysaccharide
Tregs	regulatory T cells
PDL	programmed death ligand
IL	interleukin
IFN	interferon
DC	dendritic cell
Myd	myeloid differentiation primary response
Fim	fimbrin
TNF	tumour necrosis factor
CD	cluster of differentiation
MAPK	mitogen-activated protein kinase
SILTs	solitary intestinal lymphoid tissues
ViCPS	Vi capsular polysaccharide
TLRs	Toll-like receptors
OmpD	outer membrane porin protein

Author details

Mashooq Ahmad Dar[1,2], Peerzada Tajamul Mumtaz[1], Shakil Ahmad Bhat[1], Qamar Taban[1], Shabir Ahmad Khan[1], Tufail Banday[3] and Syed Mudasir Ahmad[1*]

1 Division of Biotechnology, Faculty of Veterinary Sciences and Animal Husbandry, Shere Kashmir University of Agricultural Sciences and Technology, Kashmir, India

2 Department of Biochemistry, University of Kashmir, Kashmir, India

3 Division of Livestock Production and Management Faculty of Veterinary Sciences and Animal Husbandry, Shere Kashmir University of Agricultural Sciences and Technology, Kashmir, India

*Address all correspondence to: mudasirbio@gmail.com

References

[1] Shu-Kee E, Pusparajah P, Nurul-Syakima AM, Hooi-Leng S, Kok-Gan C, Learn-Han L. Salmonella: A review on pathogenesis, epidemiology and antibiotic resistance. Frontiers in Life Science. 2015;**8**:284-293. DOI: 10.1080/21553769.2015.1051243

[2] Andino A, Hanning I. *Salmonella enterica*: Survival, colonization, and virulence differences among serovars. The Scientific World Journal. 2015. DOI: 10.1155/2015/520179 (review article)

[3] Dar MA, Ahmad SM, Bhat SA, Ahmad R, Urwat U, Mumtaz PT, et al. Salmonella typhimurium in poultry: A review. World's Poultry Science Journal. 2017;**73**:345-354

[4] Rabsch W, Tschäpe H, Baumler AJ. Non-typhoidal salmonellosis: Emerging problems. Microbes and Infection. 2001;**3**:237-247

[5] Rodriguez A, Pangloli P, Richards HA, Mount JR, Draughon FA. Prevalence of Salmonella in diverse environmental farm samples. Journal of Food Protection. 2006;**69**:2576-2580

[6] Smith SI, Seriki A, Ajayi A. Typhoidal and non-typhoidal Salmonella infections in Africa. European Journal of Clinical Microbiology & Infectious Diseases. 2016;**35**:1913-1922

[7] Majowicz SE, Musto J, Scallan E, Angulo FJ, Kirk M, O'Brien SJ, et al. The global burden of nontyphoidal *Salmonella gastroenteritis*. Clinical Infectious Diseases. 2010;**50**:882-889

[8] Hardy A. Salmonella: A continuing problem. Postgraduate Medical Journal. 2004;**80**:541-545. DOI: 10.1136/pgmj.2003.016584

[9] Meltzer E, Schwartz E. Enteric fever: A travel medicine oriented view. Current Opinion in Infectious Diseases. 2010, 2010;**23**:432-437. DOI: 10.1097/QCO.0b013e32833c7cal

[10] Chowdhury MAJ, Shumy F, Anam AM, Chowdhury MK. Current status of typhoid fever: A review. Bangladesh Medical Journal. 2014;**43**(2)

[11] Ohad GM, Erin CB, Guntram AG. Same species, different diseases: How and why typhoidal and non-typhoidal *Salmonella enterica* serovars differ. Frontiers in Microbiology. 2014;**5**(391)

[12] Berkley JA, Lowe BS, Mwangi I, Williams T, Bauni E, Mwarumba S. Bacteremia among children admitted to a rural hospital in Kenya. The New England Journal of Medicine. 2005;**352**:39-47. DOI: 10.1056/NEJMoa040275

[13] Brent AJ, Oundo JO, Mwangi I, Ochola L, Lowe B, Berkley JA. Salmonella bacteremia in Kenyan children. The Paediatrics Infectious Disease Journal. 2006;**25**:230-236. DOI: 10.1097/01.inf.0000202066.02212

[14] Stoycheva M, Murdjeva M. Serum levels of interferon-gamma, interleukin-12, tumour necrosis factor-alpha, and interleukin-10, and bacterial clearance in patients with gastroenteric Salmonella infection. Scandinavian Journal of Infectious Diseases. 2005;**37**:11-14. DOI: 10.1080/00365540410026068

[15] De Lappe N. Salmonella Taxonomy. Version 1. Ref and research of animal salmonelloses caused by NSRLFM041. Dept of Medical Microbiology, Division of Serovars having a Public Health Importance. Clinical Microbiology, Galway University Hospitals; 2009

[16] Uzzau S, Leori GS, Petruzzi V, Watson PR, Schianchi G, Bacciu D,

et al. *Salmonella enterica* serovar-host specificity does not correlate with the magnitude of intestinal invasion in sheep. Infection and Immunity. 2001;**69**:3092-3099

[17] Wallis TS. Host-specificity of Salmonella infections in animal species. In: 'Salmonella' Infections: Clinical, Immunological and Molecular Aspects. Cambridge University Press; 2005. pp. 57-80

[18] Ellermeier CD, Slauch JM. The Genus Salmonella. In: Dworkin M, Falkow S, Rosenberg E, Schleifer KH, Stackebrandt E, editors. The Prokaryotes: A Handbook on the Biology of Bacteria. 3rd ed. Vol. 6. Springer Science and Business Media, LLC; 2006. pp. 123-158

[19] Uzzau S, Brown DJ, Wallis T, Rubino S, Leori G, Bernard S, et al. Host adapted serotypes of *Salmonella enterica*. Epidemiology and Infection. 2000;**125**:229 255

[20] Baumler AJ, Tsolis RM, Ficht TA, Adams LG. Evolution of host adaptation in *Salmonella enterica*. Infection and Immunity. 1998;**66**:4579-4587

[21] Knodler LA, Finlay BB. Salmonella and apoptosis; to live or let die? Microbes and Infection. 2001;**3**:1321-1326

[22] Rubino S, Leori G, Rizzu P, Erre G, Colombo MM, Uzzau S, et al. TnphoA Salmonella abortusovis mutants unable to adhere to epithelial cells and with reduced virulence in mice. Infection and Immunity. 1993;**61**:1786-1792

[23] Watson PR, Galyov EE, Paulin SM, Jones PW, Wallis TS. Mutation of invH, but not stn, reduces Salmonella-induced enteritis in cattle. Infection and Immunity. 1998;**30**:210-219

[24] Pan Z, Carter B, Nunez-Garcia J, Abuoun M, Fookes M, Ivens A, et al. Identification of genetic and phenotypic differences associated with prevalent and non-prevalent Salmonella enteritidis in amino acid transport. Microbiology. 2009;**155**:3200-3213

[25] Gantois I, Ducatelle R, Pasmans F, Haesebrouck F, Van Immerseel F. *Salmonella enterica* serovar Enteritidis genes induced during oviduct colonization and egg contamination in laying hens. Applied and Environmental Microbiology. 2008;**74**:6616-6622

[26] Guard J, Shah DH, Morales CA, Call DR. Evolutionary trends associated with niche specialization as modelled by whole genome analysis of egg contaminating *Salmonella enterica* serovar Enteritidis. In: Porwollik S, editor. Salmonella: From Genome to Function. San Diego, CA: Caister Academic Press; 2011. pp. 91-106

[27] Clarke RC, Gyles CL. Salmonella. In: Pathogenesis of Bacterial Infections in Animals. 2nd ed. Ames, Iowa: Iowa State University Press; 1993. pp. 133-153

[28] Chiu CH, Tang P, Chu C, Hu S, Bao Q, Yu J, et al. The genome sequence of *Salmonella enterica* serovar Choleraesuis, a highly invasive and resistant zoonotic pathogen. Nucleic Acids Research. 2005;**33**:1690-1698

[29] Kingsley RA, Msefula CL, Thomson NR, Kariuki S, Holt KE, Gordon MA, et al. Epidemic multiple drug resistant *Salmonella typhimurium* causing invasive disease in sub-Saharan Africa have a distinct genotype. Genome Research. 2009;**19**:2279-2287

[30] Thomson NR, Clayton DJ, Windhorst D, Vernikos G, Davidson S, Churcher C, et al. Comparative genome analysis of *Salmonella enteritidis* PT4 and *Salmonella gallinarum* 287/91 provides insights into evolutionary and host adaptation pathways. Genome Research. 2008;**18**:1624-1637

[31] Kisiela DI, Chattopadhyay S, Libby SJ, Karlinsey JE, Fang FC, Tchesnokova V, et al. Evolution of *Salmonella enterica* virulence via point mutations in the fimbrial adhesin. PLoS Pathogens. 2012;**8**:e1002733

[32] Olsen JE, Hoegh-Andersen KH, Casadesús J, Rosenkranzt J, Chadfield MS, Thomsen LE. The role of flagella and chemotaxis genes in host pathogen interaction of the host adapted *Salmonella enterica* serovar Dublin compared to the broad host range serovar S. Typhimurium. BMC Microbiology. 2013;**13**:67

[33] Rabsch W, Andrews HL, Kingsley RA, Prager R, Tschäpe H, Adams LG, et al. *Salmonella enterica* serotype Typhimurium and its host adapted variants. Infection and Immunity. 2002;**70**:2249-2255

[34] Heithoff DM, Shimp WR, Lau PW, Badie G, Enioutina EY, Daynes RA, et al. Human *Salmonella* clinical isolates distinct from those of animal origin. Applied and Environmental Microbiology. 2008;**74**:1757-1766

[35] Guo A, Cao S, Tu L, Chen P, Zhang C, Jia A, et al. FimH alleles direct preferential binding of Salmonella to distinct mammalian cells or to avian cells. Microbiology. 2009;**155**:1623-1633

[36] De Jong HK, Parry CM, van der Poll T, Wiersinga WJ. Host–pathogen interaction in invasive Salmonellosis. PLoS Pathogens. 2012;**8**:e1002933

[37] Eswarappa SM, Janice J, Nagarajan AG, Balasundaram SV, Karnam G, Dixit NM, et al. Differentially evolved genes of *Salmonella* pathogenicity islands: Insights into the mechanism of host specificity in *Salmonella*. PLoS One. 2008;**3**(12):e3829

[38] Eswarappa SM, Janice J, Balasundaram SV, Dixit NM, Chakravortty D. Host-specificity of *Salmonella enterica* serovar gallinarum: Insights from comparative genomics. Infection, Genetics and Evolution. 2009;**9**:468-473

[39] Liu WQ, Feng Y, Wang Y, Zou QH, Chen F, Guo JT, et al. *Salmonella paratyphi* C: Genetic divergence from *Salmonella choleraesuis* and pathogenic convergence with *Salmonella typhi*. PLoS One. 2009;**4**:e4510

[40] Scheelings TF, Lightfoot D, Holz P. Prevalence of Salmonella in Australian reptiles. Journal of Wildlife Diseases. 2011;**47**:1-11

[41] Kaiser P, Hardt WD. Salmonella typhimurium diarrhea: Switching the mucosal epithelium from homeostasis to defense. Current Opinion in Immunology. 2011;**23**:456-463

[42] Oanh HP, Stephen JM. Protective host immune responses to Salmonella infection. Future Microbiology. 2015;**10**:101-110

[43] Jones BD, Ghori N, Falkow S. Salmonella typhimurium initiates murine infection by penetrating and destroying the specialized epithelial M cells of the Peyer's patches. The Journal of Experimental Medicine. 1994;**180**:15-23

[44] Van der Velden AW, Velasquez M, Starnbach MN. Salmonella rapidly kill dendritic cells via a caspase-1-dependent mechanism. Journal of Immunology. 2003;**171**:6742-6749

[45] Bryan C, Guntram AG, Finlay BB. Salmonella, the host and disease: A brief review. Immunology and Cell Biology. 2007;**85**:112-118

[46] Hamada H, Hiroi T, Nishiyama Y, Takahashi H, Masunaga Y, Hachimura S, et al. Identification of multiple isolated lymphoid follicles on the antimesenteric wall of the mouse small intestine. Journal of Immunology. 2002;**168**:57-64

[47] Pabst O, Bernhardt G. The puzzle of intestinal lamina propria dendritic cells and macrophages. European Journal of Immunology. 2010;**40**:2107-2111

[48] Halle S, Bumann D, Herbrand H, Willer Y, Dähne S, Förster R, et al. Solitary intestinal lymphoid tissue provides a productive port of entry for *Salmonella enterica* serovar Typhimurium. Infection and Immunity. 2007;**75**:1577-1585

[49] Kraus MD, Amatya B, Kimula Y. Histopathology of typhoid enteritis: Morphologic and immunophenotypic findings. Modern Pathology. 1999;**12**:949-955

[50] Jang MH, Kweon MN, Yamamoto M, Terahara K, Sasakawa C, Suzuki T, et al. Intestinal villous M cells: An antigen entry site in the mucosal epithelium. Proceedings of the National Academy of Sciences of the United States of America. 2004;**101**:6110-6115

[51] Martinoli C, Chiavelli A, Rescigno M. Entry route of *Salmonella typhimurium* directs the type of induced immune response. Immunity. 2007;**27**:975-984

[52] Niess JH, Reinecker HC. Dendritic cells in the recognition of intestinal microbiota. Cellular Microbiology. 2006;**8**:558-564

[53] Schulz O, Jaensson E, Emma KP, Xiaosun L, Worbs T, Agace WW, et al. Intestinal CD103+, but not CX3CR1+, antigen sampling cells migrate in lymph and serve classical dendritic cell functions. The Journal of Experimental Medicine. 2009;**206**:3101-3114

[54] Persson EK, Jaensson E, Agace WW. The diverse ontogeny and function of murine small intestinal dendritic cell/macrophage subsets. Immunobiology. 2010;**215**:692-697

[55] Vazquez-Torres A, Jones-Carson J, Bäumler AJ, Falkow S, Valdivia R, Brown W, et al. Extraintestinal dissemination of Salmonella by CD18-expressing phagocytes. Nature. 1999;**401**:804-808

[56] Gerichter CB. The dissemination of *Salmonella typhi*, *S. paratyphi* A and *S. paratyphi* B through the organs of the white mouse by oral infection. The Journal of Hygiene (Lond.). 1960;**58**:307-319

[57] Griffin AJ, Li LX, Voedisch S, Pabst O, McSorley SJ. Dissemination of persistent intestinal bacteria via the mesenteric lymph nodes causes typhoid relapse. Infection and Immunity. 2001

[58] Worley MJ, Nieman GS, Geddes K, Heffron F. Salmonella typhimurium disseminates within its host by manipulating the motility of infected cells. Proceedings of the National Academy of Sciences of the United States of America. 2006;**103**:17915-17920

[59] Rescigno M, Urbano M, Valzasina B, Francolini M, Rotta G, Bonasio R, et al. Dendritic cells express tight junction proteins and penetrate gut epithelial monolayers to sample bacteria. Nature Immunology. 2001;**2**:361-367

[60] Niess JH, Brand S, Gu X, Landsman L, Jung S, McCormick BA, et al. CX3CR1-mediated dendritic cell access to the intestinal lumen and bacterial clearance. Science. 2005;**307**:254-258

[61] Vallon-Eberhard A, Landsman L, Yogev N, Verrier B, Jung S. Transepithelial pathogen uptake into the small intestinal lamina propria. Journal of Immunology. 2006;**176**:2465-2469

[62] Iwasaki A, Kelsall BL. Localization of distinct Peyer's patch dendritic cell subsets and their recruitment by chemokines macrophage inflammatory protein (MIP)-3alpha, MIP-3 beta, and secondary lymphoid organ chemokine. The

Journal of Experimental Medicine. 2000;**191**:1381-1394

[63] Carter PB, Collins FM. The route of enteric infection in normal mice. The Journal of Experimental Medicine. 1974;**139**:1189-1203

[64] McSorley SJ, Asch S, Costalonga M, Rieinhardt RL, Jenkins MK. Tracking Salmonella-specific CD4 T cells in vivo reveals a local mucosal response to a disseminated infection. Immunity. 2002;**16**:365-377

[65] Tam MA, Rydstrom A, Sundquist M, Wick MJ. Early cellular responses to Salmonella infection: Dendritic cells, monocytes, and more. Immunological Reviews. 2008;**225**:140-162

[66] Moon JJ, McSorley SJ. Tracking the dynamics of Salmonella specific T cell responses. Current Topics in Microbiology and Immunology. 2009;**334**:179-198

[67] Bonneau M, Epardaud M, Payot F, Niborski V, Thoulouze MI, Bernex F, et al. Migratory monocytes and granulocytes are major lymphatic carriers of Salmonella from tissue to draining lymph node. Journal of Leukocyte Biology. 2006;**79**:268-276

[68] Jones BD, Falkow S. Salmonellosis: Host immune responses and bacterial virulence determinants. Annual Review of Immunology. 1996;**14**:533-561

[69] Griffin AJ, McSorley SJ. Development of protective immunity to Salmonella, a mucosal pathogen with a systemic agenda. Mucosal Immunology. 2011;**4**:371-382

[70] Yu YA, Shabahang S, Timiryasova TM, Zhang Q, Beltz R, Gentschev I, et al. Visualization of tumors and metastases in live animals with bacteria and vaccinia virus encoding light-emitting proteins. Nature Biotechnology. 2004;**22**:313-320

[71] Low KB, Ittensohn M, Le T, Platt J, Sodi S, Amoss M, et al. Lipid A mutant Salmonella with suppressed virulence and TNF alpha induction retain tumor-targeting in vivo. Nature Biotechnology. 1999;**17**:37-41

[72] McSorley SJ, Jenkins MK. Antibody is required for protection against virulent but not attenuated *Salmonella enterica* serovar typhimurium. Infection and Immunity. 2000;**68**:3344-3348

[73] Sheppard M. Dynamics of bacterial growth and distribution within the liver during Salmonella infection. Cellular Microbiology. 2003;**5**:593-600

[74] Richter-Dahlfors A, Buchan AM, Finlay BB. Murine salmonellosis studied by confocal microscopy: Salmonella typhimurium resides intracellularly inside macrophages and exerts a cytotoxic effect on phagocytes in vivo. The Journal of Experimental Medicine. 1997;**186**:569-580

[75] Vazquez-Torres A, Jones-Carson J, Mastroeni P, Ischiropoulos H, Fang FC. Antimicrobial actions of the NADPH phagocyte oxidase and inducible nitric oxide synthase in experimental salmonellosis. I. Effects on microbial killing by activated peritoneal macrophages in vitro. The Journal of Experimental Medicine. 2000;**192**:227-236

[76] Chakravortty D, Hansen-Wester I, Hensel M. Salmonella Pathogenicity Island 2 mediates protection of intracellular Salmonella from reactive nitrogen intermediates. The Journal of Experimental Medicine. 2002;**195**:1155-1166

[77] Garvis SG, Beuzon CR, Holden DW. A role for the PhoP/Q regulon in inhibition of fusion between lysosomes and Salmonella-containing vacuoles in macrophages. Cellular Microbiology. 2001;**3**:731-744

[78] White JK, Mastroeni P, Popoff JF, Evans CA, Blackwell JM.

Slc11a1-mediated resistance to *Salmonella enterica* serovar Typhimurium and *Leishmania donovani* infections does not require functional inducible nitric oxide synthase or phagocyte oxidase activity. Journal of Leukocyte Biology. 2005;77:311-320

[79] Fields PI, Swanson RV, Haidaris CG, Heffron F. Mutants of *Salmonella typhimurium* that cannot survive within the macrophage are avirulent. Proceedings of the National Academy of Sciences of the United States of America. 1986;**83**:5189-5193

[80] Rydstrom A, Wick MJ. Monocyte recruitment, activation, and function in the gut-associated lymphoid tissue during oral Salmonella infection. Journal of Immunology. 2007;**178**:5789-5801

[81] Judith B, Perez-Lopez A, Sean-Paul N, Manuela R. Exploiting host immunity: The Salmonella paradigm. Trends in Immunology. 2015;**36**(2). DOI: 10.1016/j.it.2014.12.003

[82] Tumbarello M, Tacconelli E, Caponera S, Cauda R, Ortona L. The impact of bacteraemia on HIV infection. Nine years experience in a large Italian university hospital. The Journal of Infection. 1995;**31**:123-131

[83] Barton GM, Medzhitov R. Toll-like receptors and their ligands. Current Topics in Microbiology and Immunology. 2002;**270**:81-92

[84] Winter SE, Thiennimitr P, Sean-Paul N, Haneda T, Maria GW. Contribution of flagellin pattern recognition to intestinal inflammation during Salmonella enterica serotype typhimurium infection. Infection and Immunity. 2009;77:1904-1916

[85] Broz P, Newton K, Lamkanfi M, Mariathasan S, Dixit VM, Monack DM. Redundant roles for inflammasome receptors NLRP3 and NLRC4 in host defense against Salmonella. The Journal of Experimental Medicine. 2010;**207**:1745-1755

[86] McSorley SJ, Ehst BD, Yu Y, Gewirtz AT. Bacterial flagellin is an effective adjuvant for CD4 T cells in vivo. Journal of Immunology. 2002;**169**:3914

[87] Salazar-Gonzalez RM, Srinivasan A, Griffin A, Muralimohan G, James M, Rajesh ER, et al. Salmonella flagellin induces bystander activation of splenic dendritic cells and hinders bacterial replication in vivo. Journal of Immunology. 2007;**179**:6169-6175

[88] Sierro F, Dubois B, Coste A, Kaiserlian D, Kraehenbuhl JP, Sirard JC. Flagellin stimulation of intestinal epithelial cells triggers CCL20-mediated migration of dendritic cells. Proceedings of the National Academy of Sciences of the United States of America. 2001;**98**:13722-13727

[89] Salazar-Gonzalez RM, Niess JH, Zammit DJ, Ravindran R, Srinivasan A, Maxwell JR, et al. CCR6-mediated dendritic cell activation of pathogen-specific T cells in Peyer's patches. Immunity. 2006;**24**:623-632

[90] Moon JJ, Chu HH, Pepper M, McSorley SJ, Jameson SC, Kedl RM, et al. Naive CD4(+) T cell frequency varies for different epitopes and predicts repertoire diversity and response magnitude. Immunity. 2007;**27**:203-213

[91] Bumann D. In vivo visualization of bacterial colonization, antigen expression and specific T-cell induction following oral administration of live recombinant *Salmonella enterica* serovar typhimurium. Infection and Immunity. 2001;**69**:4618-4626

[92] Ravindran R, Foley J, Stoklasek T, Glimcher LH, McSorley SJ. Expression of T-bet by CD4 T cells is essential for resistance to Salmonella infection. Journal of Immunology. 2005;**175**:4603-4610

[93] McSorley SJ, Cookson BT, Jenkins MK. Characterization of CD4+ T cell responses during natural infection with *Salmonella typhimurium*. Journal of Immunology. 2000;**164**:986-993

[94] Hayashi F, Smith KD, Ozinsky A, Hawn TR, Yi EC, Goodlett DR, et al. The innate immune response to bacterial flagellin is mediated by Toll-like receptor 5. Nature. 2001;**410**:1099-1103

[95] Ravindran R, McSorley SJ. Tracking the dynamics of T-cell activation in response to Salmonella infection. Immunology. 2005;**114**:450-458

[96] Srinivasan A, McSorley SJ. Activation of Salmonella-specific immune responses in the intestinal mucosa. Archivum Immunologiae et Therapiae Experimentalis. 2006;**54**:25-31

[97] Letran SE, Lee SJ, Atif SM, Uematsu S, Akira S, McSorley SJ. TLR5 functions as an endocytic receptor to enhance flagellin-specific adaptive immunity. European Journal of Immunology. 2011;**41**:29-38

[98] Voedisch S, Koenecke C, David S, Herbrand H, Förster R, Rhen M, et al. Mesenteric lymph nodes confine dendritic cell mediated dissemination of *Salmonella enterica* serovar Typhimurium and limit systemic disease in mice. Infection and Immunity. 2009;**77**:3170-3180

[99] Monack DM, Bouley DM, Falkow S. *Salmonella typhimurium* persists within macrophages in the mesenteric lymph nodes of chronically infected Nramp1+/+ mice and can be reactivated by IFN gamma neutralization. The Journal of Experimental Medicine. 2004;**199**:231-241

[100] Sinha K, Mastroeni P, Harrison J, de Hormaeche RD, Hormaeche CE. Salmonella typhimurium aroA, htrA, and AroD htrA mutants cause progressive infections in athymic (nu/nu) BALB/c mice. Infection and Immunity. 1997;**65**:1566-1569

[101] Mittrucker HW, Raupach B, Kohler A, Kaufmann SH. Cutting edge: Role of B lymphocytes in protective immunity against *Salmonella typhimurium* infection. Journal of Immunology. 2000;**164**:1648-1652

[102] Johanns TM, Ertelt JM, Rowe JH, Way SS. Regulatory T cell suppressive potency dictates the balance between bacterial proliferation and clearance during persistent Salmonella infection. PLoS Pathogens. 2010;**6**:e1001043

[103] Srinivasan A, Foley J, McSorley SJ. Massive number of antigen specific CD4 T cells during vaccination with live attenuated Salmonella causes interclonal competition. Journal of Immunology. 2004;**172**:6884-6893

[104] Srinivasan A, McSorley SJ. Visualizing the immune response to pathogens. Current Opinion in Immunology. 2004;**16**:494-498

[105] McLachlan JB, Catron DM, Moon JJ, Jenkins MK. Dendritic cell antigen presentation drives simultaneous cytokine production by effector and regulatory T cells in inflamed skin. Immunity. 2009;**30**:277-288

[106] Tobar JA, Leandro JC, Susan MB, Pablo AG, Jorge EM, Sergio AQ, et al. Virulent *Salmonella enterica* serovar typhimurium evades adaptive immunity by preventing dendritic cells from activating T cells. Infection and Immunity. 2006;**74**:6438-6448

[107] Hess J, Ladel C, Miko D, Kaufmann SH. Salmonella typhimurium aroA-infection in gene-targeted immunodeficient mice: Major role of CD4+ TCR-alpha beta cells and IFN-gamma in bacterial clearance independent of intracellular location. Journal of Immunology. 1996;**156**:3321-3326

[108] Halici S, Zenk SF, Jantsch J, Hensel M. Functional analysis of the Salmonella pathogenicity island 2-mediated inhibition of antigen presentation in dendritic cells. Infection and Immunity. 2008;**76**:4924-4933

[109] Yrlid U, Wick MJ. Antigen presentation capacity and cytokine production by murine splenic dendritic cell subsets upon Salmonella encounter. Journal of Immunology. 2002;**169**:108-116

[110] Srinivasan A, Nanton M, Griffin A, McSorley SJ. Culling of activated CD4 T cells during typhoid is driven by Salmonella virulence genes. Journal of Immunology. 2009;**182**:7838-7845

[111] VanCott JL, Chatfield SN, Roberts M, Hone DM, Hohmann EL, Pascual DW, et al. Regulation of host immune responses by modification of Salmonella virulence genes. Nature Medicine. 1998;**4**:1247-1252

[112] Xu L, Kitani A, Strober W. Molecular mechanisms regulating TGF beta-induced Foxp3 expression. Mucosal Immunology. 2010;**3**:230-238

[113] Weaver CT, Hatton RD, Mangan PR, Harrington LE. IL-17 family cytokines and the expanding diversity of effector T cell lineages. Annual Review of Immunology. 2007;**25**:821-852

[114] Curtis MM, Way SS. Interleukin-17 in host defence against bacterial, mycobacterial and fungal pathogens. Immunology. 2009;**126**:177-185

[115] Raffatellu M, Santos RL, Verhoeven DE, George MD, Wilson RP, Winter SE, et al. Simian immunodeficiency virus-induced mucosal interleukin-17 deficiency promotes Salmonella dissemination from the gut. Nature Medicine. 2008;**14**:421-428

[116] Schulz SM, Kohler G, Holscher C, Iwakura Y, Alber G. IL-17A is produced by Th17, gamma delta T cells and other CD4- lymphocytes during infection with *Salmonella enterica* serovar enteritidis and has a mild effect in bacterial clearance. International Immunology. 2008;**20**:1129-1138

[117] Santos RL, Raffatellu M, Bevins CL, Adams LG, Tükel C, Tsolis RM, et al. Life in the inflamed intestine, Salmonella style. Trends in Microbiology. 2009;**17**:498-506

[118] MacLennan CA, Esther NG, Chisomo LM, Robert AK, Nicholas R, Thomson SA. The neglected role of antibody in protection against bacteremia caused by nontyphoidal strains of Salmonella in African children. The Journal of Clinical Investigation. 2008;**118**:1553-1562

[119] Cunningham AF, Gaspal F, Serre K, Mohr E, Henderson IR, Scott-Tucker A, et al. Salmonella induces a switched antibody response without germinal centers that impedes the extracellular spread of infection. Journal of Immunology. 2007;**178**:6200-6207

[120] Bueno SM, Gonzalez PA, Schwebach JR, Kalergis AM. T cell immunity evasion by virulent *Salmonella enterica*. Immunology Letters. 2007;**111**:14-20

[121] Barr TA, Brown S, Mastroeni P, Gray D. TLR and B cell receptor signals to B cells differentially program primary and memory Th1 responses to *Salmonella enterica*. Journal of Immunology. 2010;**185**:2783-2789

[122] Neves P, Lampropoulou V, Calderon-Gomez E, Roch T, Stervbo U, Shen P, et al. Signaling via the MyD88 adaptor protein in B cells suppresses protective immunity during *Salmonella typhimurium* infection. Immunity. 2010;**33**:777-790

[123] Wijburg OL, Uren TK, Simpfendorfer K, Johansen FE,

Brandtzaeg P, Strugnell RA. Innate secretory antibodies protect against natural *Salmonella typhimurium* infection. The Journal of Experimental Medicine. 2006;**203**:21-26

[124] Guzman CA, Borsutzky S, Griot-Wenk M, Metcalfe IC, Pearman J, Collioud A, et al. Vaccines against typhoid fever. Vaccine. 2006;**24**:3804-3811

[125] Gil-Cruz C, Bobat S, Jennifer L, Marshall RA, Kingsley EA, Ross IR. The porin OmpD from nontyphoidal Salmonella is a key target for a protective B1b cell antibody response. Proceedings of the National Academy of Sciences of the United States of America. 2009;**106**:9803-9808

Chapter 7

Application of Artificial Barrier as Mitigation of *E. coli* Which Pass through Riverbank Filtration

Nur Aziemah Abd Rashid and Ismail Abustan

Abstract

Water security in the water treatment plant has been doubted, and the treatment process may have given unreliable and unsafe water to the public. A newspaper reported on November 19, 2011, that laboratory tests on water samples in Kelantan for each year by the Ministry of Health have found harmful bacteria including *Escherichia coli* (*E. coli*) in the water samples. More worryingly, it was stated in a study that chlorine in water treated with high chlorine can be harmful to human health. In 2010, Malaysia has begun to approach a natural treatment technique, namely, riverbank filtration (RBF), and firstly used it at the Water Treatment Plant in Jeli, Kelantan, and Kuala Kangsar, Perak. RBF limitation is the invisible groundwater flow that makes it difficult to predict the transport of contaminants. Managing groundwater is important to ensure that water is aligned in compliance with government legislation and environmental protection. Due to that, this study suggests an implementation of an artificial barrier for microorganism in RBF to sustain the good water quality abstracted from the abstraction well. This pretreatment or purifying method is to improve the effectiveness of RBF in removing pollutants during shock loads and reduce the load placed in the water treatment process.

Keywords: artificial barrier, riverbank filtration, *E. coli*, groundwater, water security

1. Introduction

Potable water access globally is now under crisis, which leads to poor human health issue, affecting Malaysia as one of the countries facing this problem. The main reasons why this happens are due to climate change, deterioration of river water quality, unreliable water treatment system, and increase of population, which, at the same time, causes water shortage to occur. During dry weather conditions, further depletion of water occurs. Pertinently, climate changes make the drought season becomes longer and hotter than usual. The dam water becomes low and the river water dries up. The deterioration of river water quality in Malaysia has brought an impact to the water treatment plant due to the increase of treatment cost and maintenance. Chemicals such as PACl, alum, and others will also be increased to treat the polluted river. In the year of 2011, it was stated in a study that chlorine in water treated with high chlorine can be harmful to human health [1]. Thus, water security in the water treatment plant has been doubted, and the treatment process may have given unreliable and unsafe water to the public. Recently, *Utusan Malaysia* newspaper reported on November 19, 2011, that laboratory tests on water samples in Kelantan for each year by the Ministry of Health have found heavy metals and harmful bacteria including *Escherichia coli* (*E. coli*) in the water samples. More worryingly, *E. coli* was also found in water supplied to homes by Air Kelantan Sdn. Bhd. (AKSB). The discovery of *E. coli* in water samples in Kelantan detected by the ministry was then carried out from 2008 to 2010.

Providing reliable and safe potable water has become a human right for us. Therefore, finding a solution to these issues is highly desirable to improve the safety and reliability of potable water. In 2010, Malaysia has begun to approach a new treatment technique, namely, riverbank filtration (RBF). RBF is a method using groundwater that is expected to provide a new way to increase water intake and untapped resources in Malaysia, firstly used at the Water Treatment Plant in Jeli, Kelantan, and Kuala Kangsar, Perak. RBF is a natural system in which it involves the entry of river water into underground aquifers and is caused by hydraulic gradients, whereby water retrieval is from collector wells located at banks, at a certain distance from the river [2]. Although it is still less than 10 years in Malaysia, RBF method shows good results to reduce the use of chemicals and produces biologically stable water; the system also improves water quality by removing particles (turbidity and suspended solids), organic pollutants, microorganisms, heavy metals, and nitrogen. One previous experience in Germany shows that RBF provides a strong barrier for various pollutants and can help to ease the temperature fluctuations and concentration peaks when it is associated with spills into rivers. It also replaces and supports other treatment processes and reduces the overall costs of water treatment plant [3]. The removal of sediment, organic and inorganic compounds, and pathogens takes place during the first meters from the river in what is known as the hyporheic zone, which usually presents reducing conditions, due to high microbial activity that consumes oxygen in the water. Within this zone, there are important biochemical processes and redox reactions that affect groundwater quality [4]. In general, every stage of RBF has an environmental influence that is from the river until abstraction well.

Safe potable water is one of the implicit requisites for a healthy human population. In the existence of RBF, artificial barrier is a new efficient purifying method to maintain safer water abstraction. This study demonstrates the potential of a new application of artificial barrier to filtrate *E. coli* in water in RBF system. The artificial barrier efficiency was examined for different media ratio. Artificial barrier is a man-made vertical barrier to pretreat water abstraction intake. It is a mixture of sand (local soil), granular activated carbon (GAC), and zeolite. Generally, the individual application of coconut shell GAC and zeolite has shown great advantages in terms of characteristics, adsorption capacities, as well as their physicochemical versatility. For that reason, the idea of combining the precursors in order to make an effective filter-based adsorbent for RBF purifying process is highly recommended. Besides that, the inherited limitation of an individual precursor in water treatment process could be minimized by combining them in layered filter adsorbent as first and second barriers in RBF aquifer due to low turbidity. GAC and zeolite have high permeability which make them suitable to be applied in RBF aquifer, which requires high permeability condition as for the RBF site. However, studies on the removal of *E. coli* from actual river water using artificial barrier (GAC and zeolite) in RBF as the pretreatment or purifying process are still limited until now. Similarly, studies concerning the optimization of adsorption treatment for the studied parameter removal from river water are inadequate. Due to that, this research study is mainly focused on the treatment of actual river water from Sungai Kerian, Lubok Buntar, Kedah, via artificial barrier fixed-bed flow studies.

2. Riverbank filtration

2.1 Principle and treatment

RBF has begun to be widely used in Malaysia as to optimize the water supply. The introduction of RBF in Malaysia is started in 2010 at Jeli, Kelantan. The plants' operation has demonstrated the success of the combination of RBF (as pretreatment) and water treatment plant (as posttreatment). Most RBF in Malaysia have been applied in Kelantan areas. After calculating all the costs (not including the cost of pumps, pipes, valves, etc.), 1 m^3 of drinking water costs approximately USD 0.04, which is considered to be a competitive price for the Malaysian. The combined method has therefore proved to be both technologically and financially viable. These findings should pave the way for other municipal authorities to follow suit by introducing their own combined RBF with ultrafiltration.

RBF post water treatment has been employed dating back to the nineteenth century. During RBF, river or lake water is extracted indirectly by drawing it through the subsurface prior to use as in **Figure 1**. The extraction is accomplished by an infiltration line of well either vertical or horizontal. The well is located at a short (below 30 m) to intermediate (up to 60 m) distance from the riverbank or lake. During extraction of water, the groundwater that discharges into the river decreases, and the groundwater table near the waterline may decrease below the river water level. To ensure a satisfactory purification, the distance between the river and the extraction well should such that the travel time exceeds 30–60 days [5].

During infiltration and travel through the soil and aquifer sediments, surface water is subjected to a combination of physical and chemical and biological processes of filtration. The top few centimeters of the riverbank materials formed are a screen or filter medium that removes the suspended solids present in the water. Heavy metal, phosphorous, and hydrophobic organic compounds present in the water are removed by adsorption onto certain aquifer materials. In the presence of biomass, the organic matter is further biodegraded (initially under oxic conditions and later under anoxic conditions). The water quality in most cases is improved by dilution of the surface water source with native groundwater [6]. When a particle becomes attached to the biofilm on the sand grain, microorganism may degrade that particle. There is an interception when particles are carried by one of the streamlines closest to the sand grain and a brushing effect occurs. There is general agreement that straining, adhesion, attachment, chemical adsorption, sedimentation, and biological growth all operate to some extent.

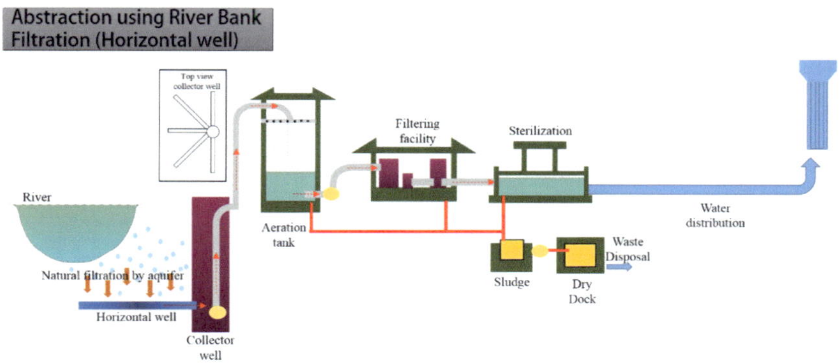

Figure 1.
Riverbank filtration system.

The conventional treatment commonly involves screening, aeration, coagulation, flocculation, sedimentation, slow sand filtration, and chlorination. The chemical treatment and waste product will increase if the pollutants in surface water increased. The RBF reduces the posttreatment step from six to only two steps which is removal of heavy metals (usually iron and manganese) by either aeration, activated carbon filter, or ultrafiltration and chlorination for taste and odor. This RBF system as a pretreatment technique applied in countries like the Netherlands, Germany, China, Korea, India, Egypt, and others has already succeeded in optimizing the potable water supply. The underground passage ensures the high quality of drinking water, which does not need any further treatment or disinfection before supply [7].

The posttreatment after RBF depends on the water abstraction water quality. Each RBF site has a different technique step for posttreatment. Previous study shows the most common pollutants that occur in RBF sites are iron and manganese. The treatments used to remove these contaminants in water are aeration, activated carbon filter, and ultrafiltration method. The second contaminant that occurs is taste and odor which are usually removed using chlorination. The third contaminant was microbiology which is solved by using ozonation and UV disinfection. This all posttreatment technique is commonly used at RBF site and summarized in **Table 1**. Meanwhile, there are RBF sites which are not using a posttreatment as a means for direct usage such as in China. However, in several years there will be oocyst problems.

2.2 Benefits and limitation

The RBF is a sustainable natural treatment process which avoids or reduces the use of chemicals and produces biologically stable water. The system improves water quality by removing particles (turbidity and suspended solid), organic pollutants,

Country	Treatment schemes	Comments
Netherland	Aeration, rapid sand filtration, activated carbon filtration and UV disinfection [8]	Electricity depends and less effective for low concentration of bacteria, virus, spores and cyst.
China	Direct usage	No iron problem. The most problem is with oocyst.
Malaysia	Cascading aerator, pressurized sand filter, ultrafiltration system [9]	Sudden increase of pollutants (cause of flood or natural disaster) may break down th ultrafiltration system and high maintenance of ultrafiltration system.
Germany	Ozonation, biological activated carbon filters, UV and safety chlorination (Small amount). [10]	The high levels of iron and manganese result to need of activated carbon filters. However, the activated carbon filters clogged. The piping get rust.
India	Aeration, filtration and chlorination. [11]	The usage of filtration as to filtrate the precipitation of iron and manganese in aeration section build a metal clogged filter. This may intribute to demenarilaziton during oxic condition.
Egypt	Aeration, filtration and chlorination [12]	-

Table 1.
Summary of RBF post treatment from other country and its limitations.

microorganism, heavy metals, and nitrogen. The RBF also helps to dampen the temperature fluctuations and concentration peaks when it is associated with spills into a river or lake. This treatment process also replaces and supports the other treatment processes by providing a robust barrier for multiple contaminants and reduces the overall cost of water treatment [3].

RBF limitation is the invisible groundwater flow that makes it difficult to predict the transport of contaminants. A specific concern of the RBF limitation is due to hydrology and dynamics of the river and groundwater, which have different climate variations (drought and rainy seasons), and thus, the groundwater level patterns result in significant fluctuation of contaminants in well stream loads. In rainy season, the rate of groundwater flow increases to a maximum level and causes small particles and pollutants to absorb into the soil where it encloses the flow along the groundwater flow, which initiates pollutants to enter the borehole. On the other hand, in dry season, minimum and ideal flow rates for pollutants are attached to the local soil. Moreover, since maximum groundwater flow rate occurs frequently in Malaysia, this incident is predicted to often result in significant fluctuations of underground hydraulic conductivity of groundwater and shock load of pollutants. Significant amount of pollutants may exist in borehole water due to high hydraulic conductivity and soil feature, which concludes that RBF is a natural treatment method that depends on natural behavior. In general, the quality of RBF water is influenced by the environmental conditions, where managing groundwater is important to ensure that water is aligned in compliance with government legislation and environmental protection.

The posttreatment step in most RBF sites is usually focused on iron and manganese treatment which result in the usage of aeration, activated carbon filter, and ultrafiltration treatment process. The weakness of this treatment which cannot be ignored has been discussed in the above section. The occurrence of the pollutants can be worse during shock load and clogging. Due to that, artificial barrier seems important which can increase the hydraulic conductivity of the underground water flow, reduce the pressure load to the aquifer during clogging, and enhance the pollutants adsorption during shock load. This can reduce the consumption of chemical treatment and strengthen the RBF barrier.

2.3 Factors influencing optimization of RBF

There are four basic important criteria affecting the performance of RBF which are hydrogeological conditions, source water quality and mixing with native groundwater, distance of the well from riverbank and spacing of wells and pumping rates, and sediment permeability. The effectiveness of RBF for removing surface water contaminants depends largely on hydrogeological conditions. It is about the soil microbiology, characteristic of the bank materials and streambed, and scouring characteristic [13]. In many countries, the alluvial soil aquifers hydraulically connected to a water course would be preferred sites for drinking water production [14]. The actual biochemical interactions that sustain the quality of the pumped bank filtration depend on numerous factors, including aquifer mineralogy and the extent of the aquifer [15].

The RBF shows a decreasing RBF water level with an increasing distance of the well apart from the riverbank. In addition to the decreasing RBF water level due to increasing distance, there is no cross flow of natural groundwater that the well could abstract river water [12]. Pumping test result shows that the water in well (below 60 m) comes from river water. However, the low-lying coastal aquifer is generally fragile and easily depleted due to anthropogenic activities and overexploitation of groundwater and agriculture. To manage and protect precious groundwater resources in a sustainable manner, the characterization and understanding of the natural evolution of groundwater chemistry are crucial to elucidate their geochemical nature and its relation.

The collector well can be far from the river if the soil type is sand and gravel such as RBF at Yellow River, China. The combination of vertical and horizontal collector well can maximize the water capacity such as RBF at Elbe River, Germany. However, clayey alluvial soil will limit the water capacity as RBF site at Lek River, Netherlands, shows the water capacity is only 0.01 MLD, compared to clayey alluvial soil at Nakdong River, Korea, which can be abstracted to 10 MLD water capacity. This shows clayey alluvial soil type needs deeper built collector well near the riverbank. The nearer to riverbank, the more water capacity can be abstracted than collector well at Nakdong River, Korea, which is only 10 MLD with 150 m distance from river, and collector well at Nile River, Egypt, with 22 MLD. Some sites do not contain gravelly sand alluvial soil type but can apply RBF such as Kali River, India. The highly pollutant river demands to use RBF methods; however, it only can abstract 0.8 MLD water capacity because the transmissivity of brownish red silty loam alluvial soil is low. Sites with clayey alluvial soil can apply limestone to increase the transmissivity of water such RBF sites at Ohio River, Kentucky, and Great Miami River, USA. Malaysia RBF sites at Sungai Semerak contain gravelly sand and shallow vertical well collector type. The shallow collector well nearer to riverbank helps RBF to avoid problem with iron and manganese. Thus, the RBF site that can supply huge water capacity is 25 MLD.

3. *Escherichia coli* in riverbank filtration

The abstracted water from RBF is very clear which has less contaminants than river water. According to previous study from other RBF sites, the contaminants that are below drinking water standard are turbidity, color, pH, TDS, chloride, ammonia, COD, BOD5, sulfate, iron, manganese, total coliform, and *E. coli*. RBF sites show great anthropogenic activity with the absence of total coliform and *E. coli* because the schmutzdecke (biofilm) layer exists at the bottom of the streamline [16] which can reduce the disinfection treatment. According to data obtained from the monitoring wells, the shallow geology of the RBF area is related to the alluvial deposition at the bottom of the streamline by the river which usually consists of upper fine, medium, and lower fine sand layers [17]. The quality of the ambient groundwater of the previous RBF sites at Louisville also shows that distance and location of the RBF wells from river are the key parameters of the RBF performance. If the RBF wells are very close to the river, then the problems of *E. coli* will be detected [18]. The existence of these enteropathogenic bacteria in abstracted well can be high in the range of 1–140 MPN/100 mL, respectively, as in **Table 2**.

Several of *E. coli* infection issues related to groundwater as drinking water were detected [19, 20] which the source of the infection was positively identified

Parameters	References				
	India [22]	China [23]	Egypt [24]	Brazil [16]	Netherland [25]
E. coli (MPN/100mL)	<140	<100	<1	Absence	10-103

***n/a = not available**

Table 2.
E. coli concentration during treated with RBF.

as a contaminated well or runoff from cow manure after torrential rain was thought to have been responsible for contamination [21]. As a safety precaution against *E. coli* infection in the body, the WHO fixed a 0.0 MPN/100 ml of *E. coli* for drinking water standard.

This study is focusing mainly on *E. coli* removal from groundwater. Typically the amount of *E. coli* depends on the aquifer types, distance of abstracted well to river, and climates. The removal of these parameters is crucial to ensure the treated groundwater can safely deliver to water treatment plant or directly distribute to consumer. *E. coli* is a Gram-negative, facultative anaerobic bacterium that belongs to the family of *Enterobacteriaceae*. *E. coli* is recognized as the most important parameter of fecal contaminants by microbiology and public health experts [26]. Depending on environmental conditions, *E. coli* can survive for 4–12 weeks [27]. There are various factors affecting the survival of *E. coli* in environment such as protozoa, antagonists, temperature, light, soil, pH, toxic substances, and oxygen [28]. The survival periods of *E. coli* in various surroundings were reported: in the groundwater at 10°C, recharged well and river water at 9–16°C, *E. coli* survived for 100 days, 63 days, and 55 days, respectively [29, 30]. Due to its strong relevance with the fecal contamination and relatively easy quantification methods, *E. coli* has been employed in a wide range of investigation including water treatment [31–33].

In natural conditions at RBF sites, water percolates through the organic soil where dissolved oxygen (DO) is consumed by the decomposition of organic matter and microbes in the soil. The decomposition process reduces the pH due to microbial action. When groundwater is pumped up to the surface, it gets into contact with air (O_2) which enters the solutions and starts the oxidation process that releases carbon dioxide (CO_2) from the groundwater to the atmosphere.

The reason for choosing *E. coli* as the main parameter is because it is a model for waterborne bacteria and reduces chemical usage in posttreatment. The *Escherichia coli* which is easily called as *E. coli* is a group of bacteria that are commonly found in food and water. Most of the *E. coli* is harmless, but some can cause sickness to human. These bacteria will lead to stomach and intestinal problems such as diarrhea and vomiting. The disease-causing *E. coli* strains live in the intestinal tracts of animals that ruminate, such as cows, deer, and goats. Bacteria early pretreatment seems important since it avoids to stimulate the bacterial growth in distribution system pipeline.

4. The possibility of *Escherichia coli* infection in riverbank filtration

The site was located at coordinates 5° 07′38.61“ N and 100° 35’44.24”, Lubok Buntar, Kedah. The examined site was influenced by the water from the Kerian River which was also influenced by the discharge of the wastewater from palm oil, mining industry, and poultry farming area at Sungai Mahang (upstream). The river water and borehole water samples were taken for laboratory (characteristics) test. **Figure 2** shows concentration plots of *E. coli* against height of water in tube well. It can be observed that the increase of height of water in tube well was caused by *E. coli* existence. The existing of *E. coli* was changed from absent to <200 MPN.

The depth of borehole was 30 m signifying that this borehole was under unconfined aquifer. The unconfined aquifer is recharged more rapidly when raining and groundwater hydraulic conductivity at maximum due to infiltration and runoff [34]. The increase of solute concentration during rainy season due to the groundwater flow exceeded the permeability of alluvial soil. Groundwater flow was maximized when raining which creates pressure to the alluvial soil. This leads small particle to flow together into abstraction well which in turn increases contaminant

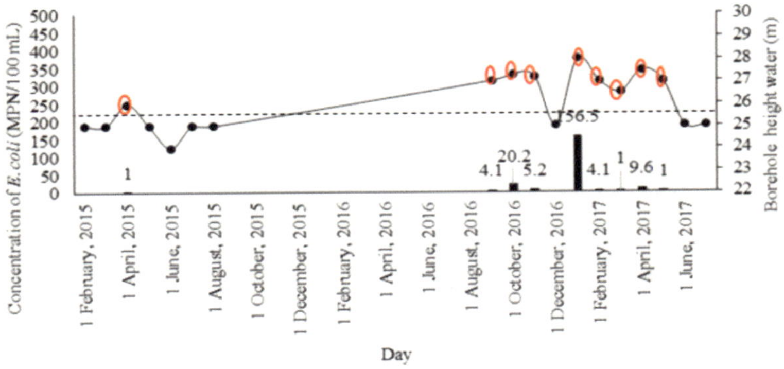

Figure 2.
The monitoring of E. coli concentration and height of borehole water for duration 2015–2017.

concentrations in abstraction water. For that reason, the application of artificial barrier seemed beneficial since it will increase the permeability of aquifer near the river avoiding small particles to flow together to abstraction well during rainy season. Besides raining, *E. coli* can penetrate into abstracted well due to pollution in streamline, abstracted well is near the riverbank, and sources of pollution such as poultry field and sanitary tank are close to abstracted well.

The experiment shows that the application of artificial barrier as RBF water purification method seems important to avoid the possibility of *E. coli* infection. Smith et al. [35] and Uhlmann et al. [36] previously identified exposure to drinking water from private underground water supply as a significant risk factor in human pathogen infections in the UK and Canada, respectively. In addition, O'Sullivan et al. [37] and Garvey et al. [38] have proposed that increases in *E. coli* infection in Ireland may be associated with water consumption from untreated water wells in rural areas, particularly following periods of excessive rainfall.

5. Artificial barrier for riverbank filtration

5.1 Methodology

The fixed-bed flow studies were carried out to evaluate their ability to remove *E. coli* during filtration process. The column was made from Perspex glass with inner diameter 8.5 cm. **Figure 3** shows a schematic diagram of the column setup used in this study. The pretreated media were filled in the column. To avoid channeling, the river water was pumped upward through the column at flow rate 50 mL/min. The flow rate was controlled by a peristaltic pump.

The water samples used in the column were taken from the Kerian River at coordinates 5° 07′38.61" N and 100° 35′44.24" E. The sand, GAC, and zeolite were oven dried for 24 hours at 105°C. Before placing the sand, GAC, and zeolite in the column, the column was washed with a solution of 3% acid nitric. The removal of *E. coli* in column test was observed in close exposure to light. This is due to the real condition in the aquifer which is close to sunlight exposure.

The *E. coli* was measured according to Method 9223B. The sample was transferred into the sterile vessel, and the water sample bottle is vigorously shaked 25 times within 7 seconds. The interval between shaking and measuring the test portion does not exceed 3 minutes. Aseptically the lid was removed, and the sample volume was adjusted to the calibrated 100 ml line of the sample container. Aseptically one packet of Colilert reagent was added to the 100 ml test bottle.

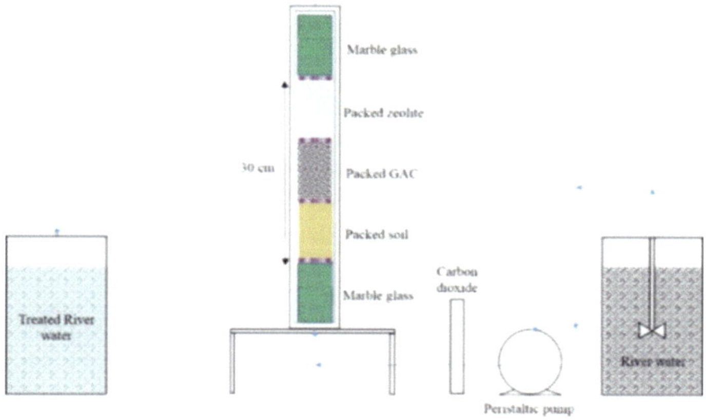

Figure 3.
Laboratory fixed bed column experimental setup.

Aseptic technique refers to a procedure that is performed under sterile conditions. The bottle was recapped and shaked until reagent was mostly dissolved. One hand was used to hold open the Quanti-Tray 2000. Well side was facing the palm of the hand. The upper part of the tray was squeezed so it bent toward the palm and gently pulled the foil tab to open the tray. Avoid touching inside of the tray or foil tab. The 100-ml sample was poured into the tray, and small wells are tapped two to three times to release air bubbles. The tray was placed with the sample into rubber insert so that the wells sat within the cutouts and rubber insert slided with tray into the sealer. The Quanti-Tray once sealed was incubated for 24 hours at 35 +/− 0.5°C. After 24 hours, the fluorescence light under UV light was counted which indicated as positive *E. coli*.

The measured *E. coli* using IDEXX was also validated with modified mTEC agar plates. Modified mTEC agar plates are prepaid powder by Arachem, BCBS2082V number. The powder was suspended in 1000 mL of distilled water for 45.6 g. The suspended powder was autoclaved and sterilized at 15 lbs. pressure (121°C) for 15 minutes. After that, the suspended powder was cooled to 45–50°C and poured into sterile petri plates. The filtered sample is placed at the top of agar and incubated at 35°C for 2 hours followed by incubation at 44.5°C for 22 hours. The modified mTEC agar contains selective and differential agents. Sodium lauryl sulfate and sodium desoxycholate are selective agents that inhibit Gram + cocci and endospore-forming bacteria. The modified mTEC agar contains the differential agent, 5-bromo-6-chloro-3-indolyl-β-D-glucuronide, which is catabolized to glucuronidase. Unlike the original mTEC method, the modified mTEC does not require the transfer of the membrane filter to another substrate. The positive colony was in magenta color. The analysis on surface morphology of the raw material was carried out using scanning electron microscope (Leo Supra 50 VP Field Emission, UK).

5.2 Result and discussion

In this study, 15 mixture components that are represented by soil, GAC, and zeolite bed height (in real site of RBF equal to distance of abstracted well water to river) were chosen for the optimization studies since they influenced the presence of *E. coli* in RBF abstracted water as well as volume of abstracted water. In addition, since the absence of *E. coli* and volume of abstracted water was concomitant, the experiments were done using high flow rate. This study determined the optimum ratio for combination of soil with GAC and zeolite that would support and improve the capability of *E. coli* removal compared to alluvial soil in RBF with a constant 50 mL/min flow rate. The removal of *E. coli* was less than 85% for soil with 81 and 82% removal as in **Figure 4**. In comparison with 70% soil combined with 15% GAC and 15% zeolite, the removal of *E. coli* was increased to 89%. Meanwhile, with 50% soil combined with 15% zeolite, the removal of *E. coli* was increased higher up to 90%. However, the combination of GAC and zeolite showed the lowest removal of *E. coli* compared to soil only by less than 50%. The honeycomb structure in GAC created the strongest biofilm layer which assisted the trap of microbe during high flow rate. Effective microbial adhesion and immobilization are essential for biofilm activities [39].

The GAC morphology (**Figure 5(a)**) showed that the surface structure and pore were well developed similar to honeycomb structure. The surface morphology of the GAC was also comparable to the analysis done by Hameed and Ahmad [40]. However, the adsorption of *E. coli* to GAC surfaces occurred on the outside of the

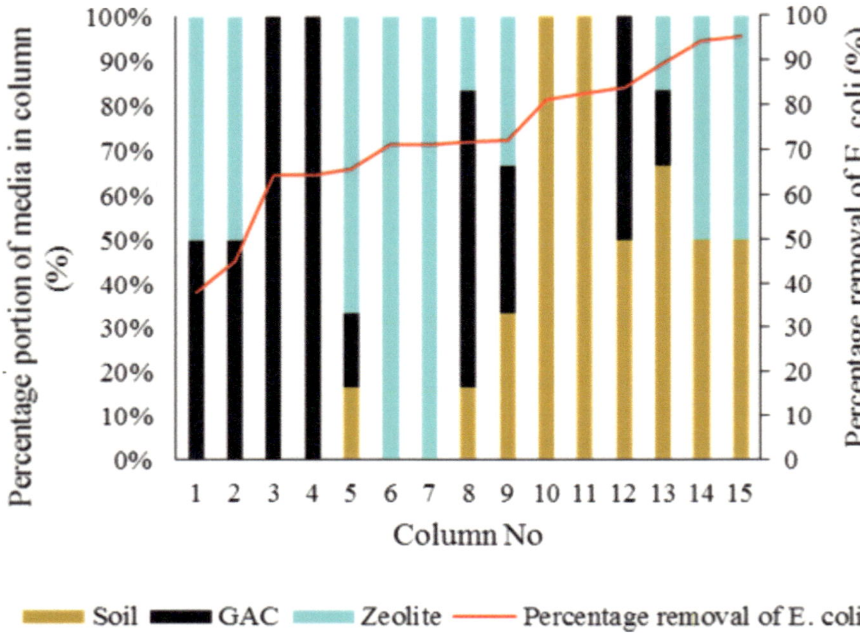

Figure 4.
Laboratory fixed bed column experimental setup.

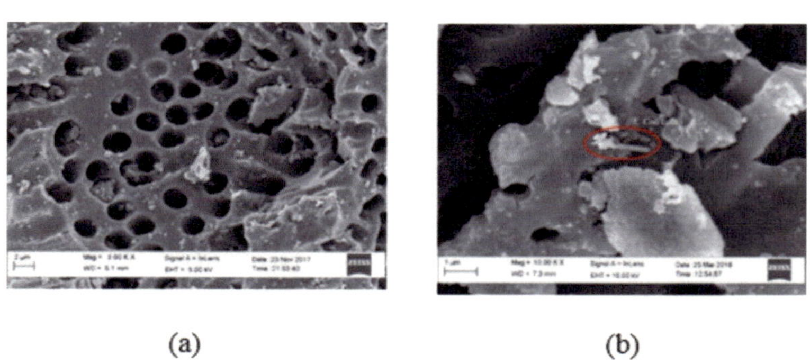

Figure 5.
The morphology of GAC for (a) before and (b) after adsorption with images of E. coli cells attach to surface.

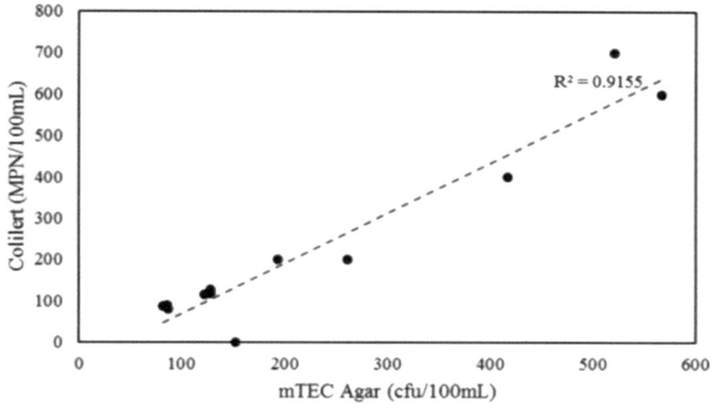

Figure 6.
Validation of measurement E. coli with using colilert and mTEC agar.

pore (honeycomb structure) as depicted in **Figure 5(b)**. *E. coli* adhesion to media surface is the initial step to schmutzdecke (biofilm) layer formation which later will create sticky surface and help in more adsorption of *E. coli*. The honeycomb structure provides strong physical confinement for the bacterial cells' adhesion and subsequently resists biofilm formation [41].

The enumeration of *E. coli* throughout optimization using Colilert. However, due to sensitivity and verification of the result, the mTEC agar enumeration method was used to increase the reliability of the result. **Figure 6** shows that the *E. coli* enumeration can be trusted due to linear R^2 of 0.92 which was acceptable (MPN acceptable values +20%). This means the results measured using mTEC agar are quite close to the mean value of MPN and in 95% of confidence limit for MPN measurement.

Until now, the health effects endemic to human for groundwater supply in Malaysia are not investigated. Casemore [42] notes that the occurrence of sporadic or pseudo-sporadic infection is particularly important in the context of groundwater-related infection. This is because the groundwater is often seen as pure quality and therefore not examined as potential sources of enteric infections that occur, thus leading to important effect.

6. Conclusion

The performance of RBF depended on alluvial soil particles' size distribution, soil gradation, and soil structure. From the monitoring, results show that the possibility of *E. coli* infection may happen. Thus, the purification method using artificial recharge seems important. In this study, the adsorption of *E. coli* by soil becomes higher in combination with GAC and zeolite. It was the honeycomb morphology of GAC that assists the attachment of *E. coli*. The schmutzdecke (biofilm) layer formation helps to enhance the *E. coli* adhesion to media surface which later will create sticky surface and help more adsorption of *E. coli*. The zeolite has higher CaO than other adsorbents; the attachment of *E. coli* in zeolite is based on mineral content. The aquifer is advisable but should not have too high or too low permeability for RBF because majority of removal mechanism was assisted by medium filter media permeability. The chemical usage technique in controlling *E. coli* in water treatment may not be a suitable method, whereby in a certain time, *E. coli* may resist to that chemical. Thus, from that reasoning, it's better to use the adsorption method.

Acknowledgements

The authors would like to acknowledge the Ministry of Education Malaysia for providing LRGS Grant on Water Security entitled Protection of Drinking Water: Source Abstraction and Treatment (203/PKT/6720006).

Author details

Nur Aziemah Abd Rashid* and Ismail Abustan
Universiti Sains Malaysia, Nibong Tebal, Malaysia

*Address all correspondence to: nuraziemahabdrashid@gmail.com

References

[1] Bull RJ, Reckhow DA, Li X, Humpage AR, Joll C, Hrudey SE. Potential carcinogenic hazards of non-regulated disinfection by-products: Haloquinones, halo-cyclopentene and cyclohexene derivatives, N-halamines, halonitriles, and heterocyclic amines. Toxicology. 2011;**286**:1-19. DOI: 10.1016/j.tox.2011.05.004

[2] Michael S. Systematic comparison of riverbank filtration sites in Austria and India [Doctoral Dissertation]. Austria: Universität Innsbruck; 2006

[3] Ray C, Grischeck T, Schubert J, Wang JZ, Speth TF. A perspective of riverbank filtration. Journal of the American Water Works Association. 2002;**94**:149-160. DOI: 10.1002/j.1551-8833.2002.tb09459

[4] Lewandowski JA, Putschew A,Schwesig D, Neumann C, Radke M. Fate of organic micropollutants in the hyporheic zone of a eutrophic lowland stream: Results of a preliminary field study. Journal of Science Total Environment. 2011;**409**:1824-1835. DOI: 10.1016/j.scitotenv.2011.01.028

[5] Huisman L, Olsthoorn TN. Artificial Groundwater Recharge. Boston: Pitman; 1983

[6] Gina M. Riverbank Filtration: The Future is Now. USA: National Water Research Institute; 2003

[7] Tischendorf W. Groundwater management for the city of Graz. In Proceedings of IWA regional conference on groundwater management in the Danube River basin and other large river basins. Belgrade: Serbia; 2007

[8] Juhasz-Holterman MHA, Peters JH, Geerts JJGM. Artificial recharge of lake excavated for gravel extraction. In: Peter et al., editors. Artificial Recharge of Groundwater. The Netherland: Balkema, Rotterdam; 1998

[9] Chew CM, David Ng KM, Richard Ooi HH, Ismail WMZW. Malaysia's largest river bank filtration and ultrafiltration systems for municipal drinking water production. Journal of Water Practice and Technology. 2015;**10**:59-65. DOI: 10.2166/wpt.2015.008

[10] Nodler K, Hillebrand O, Idzik K, Strathmann M, Schiperski F, Zirlewagen J, et al. Occurrence and fate of the angiotensin II receptor antagonist transformation product valsartan acid in water cycle—A comparative study with selected β-blockers and the persistent anthropogenic wastewater indicators carbamazepine and acesulfame. Journal of Water Research. 2013;**47**:6650-6659. DOI: 10.1016/j.watres.2013.08.034

[11] Singh P, Kumar P, Mehrotra I, Grischek T. Impact of riverbank filtration on treatment of polluted river water. Journal of Environmental Management. 2009;**91**:1055-1062. DOI: 10.1016/j.jenvman.2009.11.013

[12] Shamrukh M, Ahmed AW. Water pollution and riverbank filtration for water supply along river Nile, Egypt. Riverbank Filtration for Water Security in Desert Countries. 2011;**233**:1824-1835. DOI: 10.1007/978-94-007-0026-0_2

[13] Sahoo GB, Ray C, Wanf JZ, Hubbs SA, Song R, Jasperse J, et al. Use of artificial neural networks to evaluate the effectiveness of riverbank filtration. Water Research. 2005;**39**:2505-2516. DOI: 10.1016/j.watres.2005.04.020

[14] Doussan C, Poitevin G, Ledoux E, Detay M. River bank filtration: modeling of the changes in water chemistry with emphasis on nitrogen species. Journal of Contaminant

Hydrology. 1997. DOI: 10.1016/S0169-7722(96)00024-1

[15] Hiscock KM, Grischeck T. Attenuation of groundwater pollution by bank filtration. Journal of Hydrology. 2002;**266**:139-144. DOI: 10.1016/S0022-1694(02)00158-0

[16] Freitas DA, Cabral JJSP, Paiva ALR, Molica RJR. Application of bank filtration technology for water quality improvement in a warm climate: A case study at Beberibe River in Brazil. Journal of Water Supply: Research and Technology. 2012;**61**:319-330. DOI: 10.2166/aqua.2012.097

[17] Lee JH, Hamm SY, Cheong JY, Kim HS, Ko EJ, Lee KS, et al. Characterizing riverbank-filtered water and river water qualities at a site in the lower Nakdong River basin, Republic of Korea. Journal of Hydrology. 2009;**376**:209-220. DOI: 10.1016/j.jhydrol.2009.07.030

[18] Wang J. Riverbank filtration case study at Louisville, Kentucky. Journal of Water Science and Technology. 2002;**43**(3):117-145. DOI: 10.1007/0-306-48154-5_8

[19] Schets FM, During M, Italiaander R, et al. Escherichia coli O157:H7 in drinking water from private water supplies in the Netherlands. Water Research. 2005;**39**(18):4485-4493

[20] Fong TT, Mansfield LS, Wilson DL, et al. Massive microbiological groundwater contamination associated with a waterborne outbreak in Lake Erie, South Bass Island, Ohio. Environmental Health Perspectives. 2007;**115**(6):856-864

[21] Charatan F. New York outbreak of E. coli poisoning affects 1000 and kills two. British Medical Journal. 1999;**319**:873

[22] Cady P, Boving B, Choudri BS, Cording A, Patil K, Reddy V. Attenuation of bacteria at a riverbank filtration site in rural India. Journal of Water Environment Research. 2014;**85**:2164-2174. DOI: 10.2175/106143013X13736496909428

[23] Hu B, Teng Y, Zhai Y, Zuo R, Li J, Chen H. Riverbank filtration in China: A review and perspective. Journal of Hydrology. 2016;**541**:914-927. DOI: 10.1016/j.jhydrol.2016.08.004

[24] Abdalla F, Shamrukh M. Riverbank filtration: Developing countries choice for water supply treatment, Egypt case. In: The 1st IWA Malaysia Young Water Professionals Conference (IWAYP2010), 1-4 March. Kuala Lumpur, Malaysia; 2010. p. 2010

[25] Enrico H, Pieter JS, Janek G, Harrie T, Gudrun M. The fate of organic micropollutants during long-term/long-distance river bank filtration. Journal of Science of the Total Environment. 2016;545-546, 629-640. DOI: 10.1016/j.scitotenv.2015.12.057

[26] Bartram J, Cotruvo J, Exner M, Fricker C, Glasmacher A. Heterotrophic plate count measurement in drinking water safety management—Report of an Expert Meeting Geneva. International Journal of Food Microbiology. 2002;**92**:241-247. DOI: 10.1016/j.ijfoodmicro.2003.08.005

[27] Edberg SC, Rice EW, Karlin RJ, Allen MJ. Escherichia coli: The best biological drinking water indicator for public health protection. Journal of Applied Microbiology. 2000

[28] Foppen JWA, Schijven JF. Evaluation of data from the literature on the transport and survival of Escherichia coli and thermotolerant coliforms in aquifers under saturated conditions. Water Research.

2006;**40**:401-426. DOI: 10.1016/j.watres.2005.11.018

[29] Goldshmi MG, Pantsili VD. Device for carving out spacing nets as series of circles. Zavodskaya Laboratoriya. 1972;(1):117

[30] Grabow WOK, Prozesky OW, Burger JS. Behavior in a river and dam of coliform bacteria with transferable or non-transferable drug-resistance. Water Research. 1975;**9**(9):777-782

[31] Bielefeldt AR, Kowalski K, Summers RS. Bacterial treatment effectiveness of point-of-use ceramic water filters. Water Research. 2009;**43**(14):3559-3565

[32] Lutterodt G, Foppen JWA, Maksoud A, Uhlenbrook S. Transport of Escherichia coli in 25 m quartz sand column. Journal of Contaminant Hydrology. 2011;**119**(1-4):80-88

[33] Sinton LW, Mackenzie ML, Karki N, Dann RL, Pang L, Close ME. Transport of Escherichia coli and F-RNA bacteriophages in a 5-M column of saturated heterogenous gravel. Water, Air, & Soil Pollution. 2012;**223**:2347-2360. DOI: 10.1007/s11270-011-1029-9

[34] Zhang G, Feng G, Li X, Xie C, Pi X. Flood effect on groundwater recharge on a typical silt loam soil. Water. 2017;**9**:1-15. DOI: 10.3390/w9070523

[35] Smith A, Reacher M, Smerdon W, et al. Outbreaks of waterborne infectious intestinal disease in England and Wales, 1992-2003. Epidemiology and Infection. 2006;**134**(6):1141-1149

[36] Uhlmann S, Galanis E, Takaro T, et al. Where's the pump? Associating sporadic enteric disease with drinking water using a geographic information system, in British Columbia, Canada, 1996-2005. Journal of Water and Health. 2009;**07**(4):692-698

[37] O'Sullivan MB, Garvey P, O'Riordan M, et al. Increase in VTEC cases in the south of Ireland: Link to private wells? Euro Surveillance. 2008;**13**(39):1-2

[38] Garvey P, McKeown P, Carroll A, et al. Epidemiology of verotoxigenic *E. coli* in Ireland, 2008. Epi Insight. 2009;**10**(9):1-10

[39] Zhu IX, Brian JB. Conventional media filtration with biological activities. In: Walid E, Rezaul K, editors. Water Treatment. Chowdhury: IntechOpen; 2013. DOI: org/10.5772/50481

[40] Hameed BH, Ahmad AA. Batch adsorption of methylene blue from aqueous solution by garlic peel, an agricultural waste biomass. Journal of Hazardous Materials. 2009;**164**(2-3):870-875. DOI: 10.1016/j.jhazmat.2008.08.084

[41] Meng Y, Yonghui D, Xiang G, Yang L. Control of bacterial adhesion and growth on honeycomb-like patterned surfaces. Colloids and Surfaces B. 2015;**135**(2015):549-555

[42] Casemore D. Towards a US national estimate of the risk of endemic waterborne disease—Sero-epidemiologic studies. Journal of Water and Health. 2006;**4**(Suppl. 2):121-164

Chapter 8

Prologue: *Escherichia coli*, *Listeria*, and *Salmonella*

Maria Teresa Mascellino

1. Introduction

The present book deals with the following microorganisms: *E. coli*, *Salmonella*, and *Listeria*. The first two are Gram-negative bacteria belonging to the group of Enterobacteriaceae with the characteristic of becoming resistant to the most common antibiotics; whereas, the last one is a Gram-positive bacterium belonging to *Corynebacterium*, *Erysipelothrix*, and other Gram-positive microorganisms showing an involvement in pathologies as newborn meningitis and gynecological infection which may interfere with the pregnancy outcome. The peculiarity of all these bacteria is that they can be transmitted by contaminated food.

2. *E. coli*

Scientific classification
Domain: Prokaryota
Kingdom: Bacteria
Phylum: Proteobacteria
Class: Gamma Proteobacteria
Order: Enterobacteriales
Family: Enterobacteriaceae
Species: *E. coli*

The bacteria, in fact, can be found in the gastrointestinal tract (GI) of humans and animals, but they are mainly considered as ubiquitous microorganisms.

This bacterium includes a single species (*E. coli*) and is divided into 171 serotypes, aerobic-anaerobic Gram-negative rods with flagella fimbriae, and able to ferment glucose and lactose.

The most important serotype is *Escherichia coli* O157:H7 or enterohemorrhagic *Escherichia coli* (EHEC), which often leads to enterohemorrhagic diarrhea and is also able to induce hemolytic uremic syndrome (HUS) which is characterized by acute renal failure, hemolytic anemia, and thrombocytopenia that are more common in children and in elderly people [1].

Serotype O157-H7 causes numerous outbreaks and sporadic cases of bloody diarrhea. Foodborne pathogenic E. coli contamination, such as that with *E. coli* O157 and O104, is very common even in developed countries. Bacterial contamination may occur from environmental, animal, or human sources and cause foodborne illness [2].

The three main diseases, depending on each particular serotype involved, are urinary tract infections, intestinal diseases, and neonatal meningitis [3].

Many different mechanisms of action are reported regarding the virulence of *E. coli*. Although most strains are saprophytic colonizing the large bowel, some types of them are involved in different pathologies such as traveler's and childhood diarrhea (ETEC and EPEC also in Mexico and North Africa EAEC), hemorrhagic colitis (EHEH), and a Shiga-like disease (EIEC). As far as this last point is concerned, it is reported that the differentiation between *Shigella* and *E. coli* is quite more complicated when we consider enteroinvasive *E. coli* (EIEC). In fact, EIEC are strains that are similar to *E. coli* but are able to cause dysentery using the same method of invasion as *Shigella*. In fact, in this specific situation, EIEC is more related to *Shigella* than to non-invasive *E. coli* [4]. This strain is among the most common cause of foodborne diseases other than of neurological and renal complications, especially in children.

Escherichia coli K1 strains are major causative agents of invasive disease of newborn infants. Colonization of the small intestine following oral administration of K1 bacteria leads rapidly to blood stream infections (BSI). Indeed, these microorganisms are the cause of life-threatening infections that are acquired from the mother at birth thus colonizing the small intestine, from where they invade the blood and central nervous system.

E. coli is increasingly present as a MDR (multi-drug resistant) bacterium, in fact its genomic outfit has acquired various antibiotic resistances through the production of ESBL [5] and carbapenemases as well as metallo-beta lactamases (NDM = New Delhi metallo-beta lactamases) making the infections of this bacterium extremely worrying [6] (**Figures 1** and **2**).

3. *Listeria monocytogenes*

Class: Bacilli
Kingdom: Bacteria
Family: Listeriaceae
Classification: *Listeria*

Listeria monocytogenes is a Gram-positive, mobile, rod-shaped bacterium that is ubiquitous in the environment. It can be isolated in soil and wood and decays in the natural environment; however, the principal acquisition of *Listeria* is through the ingestion of contaminated food products. *Listeria* is a foodborne pathogen that contaminates food-processing environments and persists within biofilms in the surroundings. The peculiar characteristic of this microorganism is its ability to grow even in extreme situations, such as under high salt conditions and refrigeration temperatures, maintaining its vitality in various food products [7]. Even though the incidence of listeriosis is lower than other enteric illnesses, infections caused by *L. monocytogenes* are more serious and may lead to hospitalizations and fatalities. These infections mainly affect women and children who acquire the disease

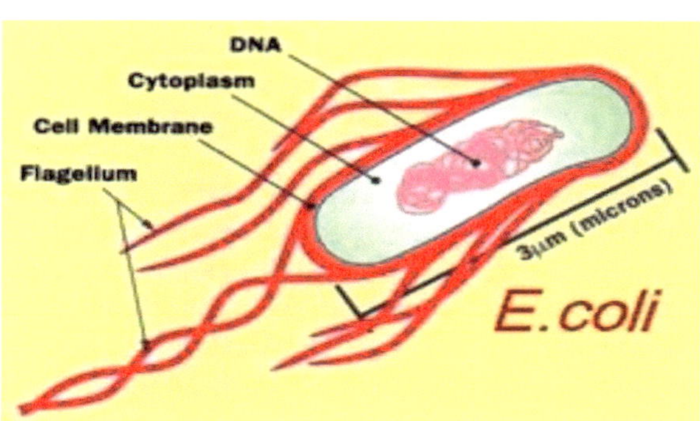

Figure 1.
Morphology of E. coli. *http://www.lacolonscopia.it/colonscopia/escherichia-coli-come-prevenirlo-e-curarlo/*

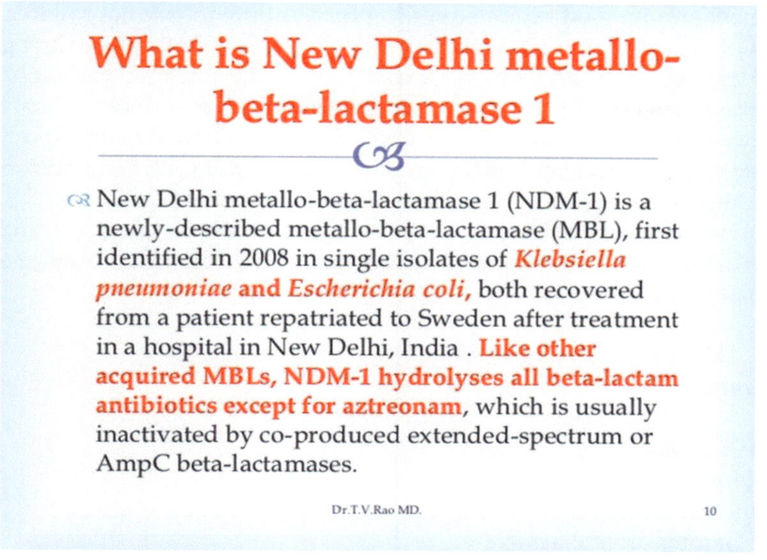

Figure 2.
Slide from "New Delhi metallo-beta-lactamase (NDM-1). Facts, controversies, solutions. An update" T.V. Rao (Powerpoint 2016). https://www.slideshare.net/doctorrao/new-delhi-metallobetalactamse

through vertical transmission from mother to infant during pregnancy or childbirth. Nosocomial infections between children are rare but anyhow they were reported. The most important disease for the newborns is the neonatal meningitis, which shows a high degree of mortality (higher in the developing countries which can reach 40–58% of cases). Listeriosis requires rapid treatment with antibiotics and most drugs suitable for Gram-positive bacteria are effective against *L. monocytogenes*. Generally, the *Listeria* clinical strains are susceptible to the common antibiotics because only a minority results as being resistant to antimicrobial agents. In the same way, several

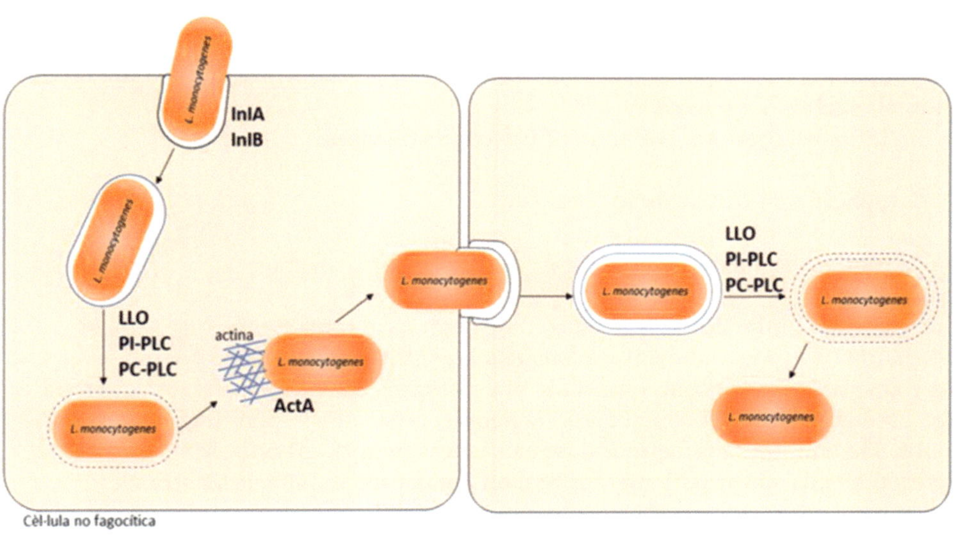

Figure 3.
Phagocytosis of Listeria. Legenda: (internalins InlA and InlB), phagosome lysis (listeriolysin O (LLO)), phosphatidylinositol-specific phospholipase C (PI-PLC) and phosphatidylcholine ((PC)-PLC), cell-to-cell spread (actin assembly-inducing protein (ActA)), intracellular growth (hexose-6-phosphate transporter (Hpt)) [10].

strains detected from food exhibited resistance to antimicrobials not suitable against listeriosis [8]. Pregnant women can carry *Listeria* asymptomatically in their gastrointestinal tract or vagina and the risk of transmitting this infection to their babies is high. The consequence of listeriosis to human health is a very important issue due to its virulence mainly in children with an underlying immunodeficiency. Symptoms include fever, headache, abdominal pain, diarrhea, vomiting, and convulsions. The complications can be appendicitis and Meckel's diverticulitis [9].

Listeria which is saprophyte in the environments such as water, soil, and food, once internalizes into the mammalian host, shows its virulence through the expression of many gene products reported in **Figure 3** [10].

4. *Salmonella*

Domain: Prokaryota
Kingdom: Bacteria
Phylum: Proteobacteria
Class: Gammaproteobacteria
Order: Enterobacteriales
Family: Enterobacteriaceae
Genre: *Salmonella*

Salmonella is the most commonly isolated bacterial agent of foodborne and epidemic infections. It was reported for the first time in 1886, in a case of swine fever by the American doctor Daniel Elmer Salmon.

The genus *Salmonella* is characterized by Gram-negative facultative anaerobic bacilli without spores. They are mobile through peritrichous flagella with the exception of *S. gallinarum* and *S. pullorum*. The serotypes are diversified according to the somatic antigen "O," the flagellar antigen "H" and the surface antigen "Vi." The Vi antigen is exclusively expressed by *S. typhi* and is able to circumvent the innate immune response by repressing flagellin and LPS expression [11]. The "O" antigens are distinguished in the serogroups A, B, C1, C2, D, and E.

Salmonella is present in the environment and can be either commensal or pathogen for men and various animals; some serotypes are exclusively pathogen for humans (i.e., *S. typhi* and *S. paratyphi* A and C), others infect both humans and animals such as *S. typhimurium* [12].

In humans, there are two kind of infectious diseases:

1. typhoid and paratyphoid fever [13]

2. minor salmonellosis [14]

Salmonella infection is transmitted through fecal route by the ingestion of contaminated food and drink. *Salmonella typhi* is responsible for typhoid fever, and its transmission can occur, especially in developing countries, by water and food infected or with direct contact among people, especially in poor hygienic conditions. The minimum infectious dose can be less than 15–20 cells. Individual sensitivity depends on the patients' age and on the nature of *Salmonella* strains.

In most cases, *Salmonella* infection occurs in mild form and resolves on its own within a few days. In these situations, the advice is not to consider the diarrheal phenomenon, since it is the natural defense mechanism used by the organism to expel germs. Normally, for *Salmonella*, it should be enough to adopt a supportive therapy: administration of oral rehydration solutions (which are used to compensate for water and salts lost with vomiting and diarrhea), lactic ferments, and probiotics.

Although salmonellosis is a bacterial infection, the use of antibiotics is not recommended as it could lengthen the persistence time of *Salmonella* in feces or induce antimicrobials resistance [15]. Hospitalization and the use of antibiotics are indicated only in severe cases (with extra-intestinal symptoms), in infants under 3 months and in subjects with chronic-degenerative diseases.

In recent times, *Salmonella* has changed its characteristics worldwide, becoming the etiologic agent of many peculiar pathological processes such as cancer development, inflammatory process, and immune-pathogenesis [16, 17] (**Figure 4**).

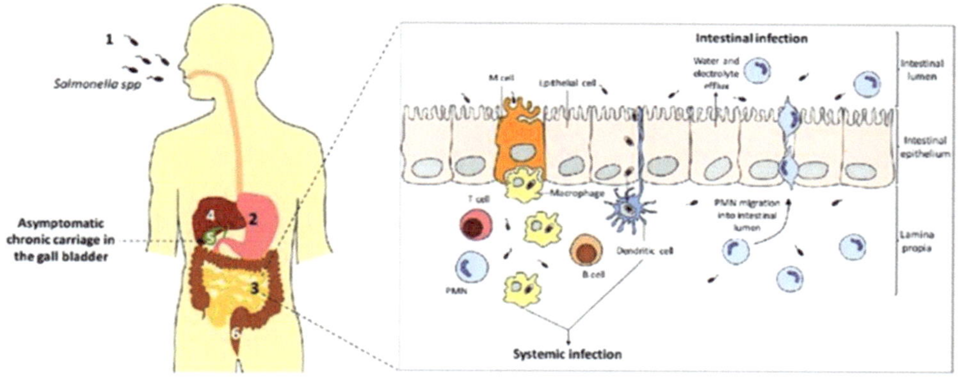

Figure 4.
Salmonella *infection pathogenesis. The ingestion of contaminated food or water begins the infective processes (gastroenteritis or systemic infection) depending on the species of* Salmonella *involved (minor and major Salmonellae). The microorganisms reach the intestinal epithelial cells and migrate to the lamina propria invading the liver from where* Salmonella *reaches the gall bladder and can cause chronic carriage which gives rise to healthy carriers [18].*

Author details

Maria Teresa Mascellino
Sapienza University of Rome, Italy

*Address all correspondence to: mariateresa.mascellino@uniroma1.it

References

[1] Tapader R, Bose D, Pal A. YghJ, the secreted metalloprotease of pathogenic *E. coli* induces hemorrhagic fluid accumulation in mouse ileal loop. Microbial Pathogenesis. 2017;**105**:96-99. DOI: 10.1016/j.micpath.2017.02.020. Epub: February 16, 2017

[2] Yang SC, Lin CH, Aljuffali IA, Fang JY. Current pathogenic *Escherichia coli* foodborne outbreak cases and therapy development. Archives of Microbiology. 2017;**199**(6):811-825. DOI: 10.1007/s00203-017-1393-y. [Epub: June 9, 2017]

[3] Daga AP, Koga VL, Soncini JGM, de Matos CM, Perugini MRE, Pelisson M, et al. *Escherichia coli* bloodstream infections in patients at a University Hospital: Virulence factors and clinical characteristics. Frontiers in Cellular and Infection Microbiology. 2019;**9**:191-201. DOI: 10.3389/fcimb.2019

[4] van den Beld MJC, Reubsaet FAG. Differentiation between *Shigella*, enteroinvasive, *Escherichia coli* (EIEC) and noninvasive *Escherichia coli*. European Journal of Clinical Microbiology & Infectious Diseases. 2012;**31**:899. DOI: 10.1007/s10096-011-1395-7

[5] Picozzi CM, Casellato S, Rossini M, Paola G, Tejada M, Costa E, et al. Extended-spectrum beta-lactamase-positive *Escherichia coli* causing complicated upper urinary tract infection: Urologist should act in time. Urology Annals. 2014;**6**(2):107-112. DOI: 10.4103/0974-7796.130536

[6] Solé M, Pitart C, Roca I, Fàbrega A, Salvador P, Muñoz L, et al. First description of an *Escherichia coli* strain producing NDM-1 Carbapenemase in Spain. Antimicrobial Agents and Chemotherapy. 2011;**55**(9):4402-4404. DOI: 10.1128/AAC.00642-11

[7] Camargo AC, Woodward JJ, Call DR, Nero LA. *Listeria monocytogenes* in food-processing facilities, food contamination, and human listeriosis: The Brazilian scenario. Foodborne Pathogens and Disease. 2017;**14**(11):623-636. DOI: 10.1089/fpd.2016.2274. Epub: 2017

[8] Radoshevich L, Cossart P. *Listeria monocytogenes*: Towards a complete picture of its physiology and pathogenesis. Nature Reviews. Microbiology. 2018;**16**(1):32-46. DOI: 10.1038/nrmicro.2017.126. [Epub: November 27, 2017]. Review

[9] Li MH, Li YJ, Hu B, Guo LY, Guo X, Guan HZ, et al. Clinical characteristics and next generation sequencing of three cases of *Listeria monocytogenes* meningitis with complications. Zhonghua Er Ke Za Zhi. 2019;**57**(8): 603-607. DOI: 10.3760/cma.j.issn.0578-1310.2019.08.007

[10] Freitag NE, Port GC, Miner MD. *Listeria monocytogenes*—From saprophyte to intracellular pathogen. Nature Reviews. Microbiology. 2009;**7**(9): 623-628. DOI: 10.1038/nrmicro2171. [Epub: August 3, 2009]

[11] de Jong HK, Parry CM, van der Poll T, Wiersinga WJ. Host–pathogen interaction in invasive salmonellosis. PLoS Pathogens. 2012;**8**(10):e1002933. DOI: 10.1371/journal.ppat.1002933. [Epub: October 4, 2012]. Review

[12] Johnson R, Ravenhall M, Pickard D, Dougan G, Byrne A, Frankel G. Comparison of *Salmonella enterica* serovars *Typhi* and *Typhimurium* reveals typhoidal serovar-specific responses to bile. Infection and Immunity. 2018;**86**(3):pii: e00490-pii: e00417. DOI: 10.1128/IAI.00490-17. Print: March 2018

[13] Johnson R, Mylona E, Frankel G. Typhoidal *Salmonella*: Distinctive

virulence factors and pathogenesis. Cellular Microbiology. 2018;**20**(9):e12939. DOI: 10.1111/cmi.12939. [Epub: August 9, 2018]. Review

[14] Fàbrega A. *Salmonella enterica* serovar *Typhimurium* skills to succeed in the host: Virulence and regulation. Clinical Microbiology Reviews. 2013;**26**(2):308-341. DOI: 10.1128/CMR.00066-12

[15] Liu S, Kilonzo-Ntheng A. Prevalence of multidrug-resistant bacteria from US-grown and imported fresh produce retailed in chain supermarkets and ethnic stores of Davidson County, Tennessee. Journal of Food Protection. 2017;**80**(3):506-514. DOI: 10.4315/0362-028X.JFP-16-178

[16] Wang CZ, Kazmierczak RA, Eisenstark A. Strains, mechanism, and perspective: Salmonella-based cancer therapy. International Journal of Microbiology. 2016;**2016**:5678702. DOI: 10.1155/2016/5678702. Review

[17] Nieto PA, Pardo-Roa C, Salazar-Echegarai FJ, Tobar HE, Coronado-Arrázola I, Riedel CA, et al. New insights about excisable pathogenicity islands in *Salmonella* and their contribution to virulence. Microbes and Infection. 2016;**18**(5):302-309. DOI: 10.1016/j.micinf.2016.02.001. [Epub: March 3, 2016]

[18] Urdaneta V, Casadesús J. Interactions between bacteria and bile salts in the gastrointestinal and hepatobiliary tracts. Frontiers in Medicine (Lausanne). 2017;**4**:163. DOI: 10.3389/fmed.2017.00163. eCollection 2017

Chapter 9

Lateral Flow Assay for *Salmonella* Detection and Potential Reagents

Dilek ÇAM

Abstract

Salmonella is among the very important pathogens threating human and animal health. It is a common food pathogen transmitted from animals to humans via contaminated food, drinking water, and air. It invades the intestinal tract of hosts and causes salmonellosis leading to death. *S. enteritidis* was the most common species accounted for all salmonellosis cases. *S. typhimurium* is also another significant species causing the serious cases worldwide. To ensure public health, early detection of pathogens is crucial. Lateral flow assay (LFA), immunochromatographic assay, is a simple and rapid diagnostic test kits used in various fields and can be developed by, aptamers, antibodies (Abs), and nucleic acids. They are also being continued to develop different capture reagents coming from the recombinant technology. It has many advantages such as having mature technology, market presence, low cost, easy to use for end users without education, and stable shelf life. Gold nanoparticles (GNPs) are the most commonly used labels in the LFAs for the naked-eye analysis. Therefore, *Salmonella* detection by LFA based on GNPs in a rapid and simple way is always open to be developed by new reagents and methods.

Keywords: *Salmonella*, gold nanoparticles, lateral flow, food pathogens, rapid detection

1. Introduction

Most of *Salmonella* infections are typically food-borne illness. It was reported that around 15% of salmonellosis cases is caused by pork [1], turkey products, and meat [2]. Early detection of pathogens which contaminated the foods or consumption products is a crucial issue especially for the government authorities to ensure public health. Thus, many kinds of identification methods are in use, and new detection platforms are also being tried to develop for improving the sensitivity and selectivity of detection with low cost as rapid tests.

Traditionally, the *Salmonella* diagnosis in the laboratory is based on common cultural techniques [3], biochemical and serological confirmation tests. Along with immunomagnetic nanospheres as immunological tools [4], multiplex PCR [5] and real-time multiplex PCR [6–9] are other detection methods of *Salmonella* in chicken samples or other sources. However, some of those techniques require 5 or 7 days, skilled personnel, sterile working conditions, and sensitive and costly equipment, and they are inconvenient for food sector or industrial applications [10] and not portable to perform sensitive and rapid microbial analysis. To develop the fast and sensitive method for bacterial antigens, electrochemical [11], optical [12], microfluidic [13], and magnetoelastic biosensors are also being developed for the detection of *Salmonella* species. Among those techniques lateral flow assay (LFA) is still the most practical and easy to use test and multiple detection tool as an immunosensor for end users.

2. Lateral flow assay

LFA, immunochromatographic strip test, which can be developed by Abs, aptamer, and nucleic acids, was described in the 1960s [14] and become a popular platform for rapid immunoassays since the mid-1980s [15–17]. Depending on their formats, LFAs might be expressed as dipstick assay, lateral flow device (LFD), point of care (POC) to bedside test, and lateral flow immunochromatographic assay (LFIA). LFAs are used to detect the presence or absence of a target analyte in sample and allow naked-eye analyses based on accumulation concepts [18]. LFAs have many advantages compared to other detection methods. They are established mature technology, with processes already developed, relative ease of manufacture, and stable shelf lives of 12–24 months often without refrigeration; easily scalable to high-volume production; and integrated with various systems, having high sensitivity, specificity, relatively low cost, market presence, and minimal education required for users and regulators [19]. However, test-to-test reproducibility, unclear patent situation, sensitivity issues in some systems, and integration with onboard electronics are drawbacks of LFAs. To note LFA market is expected to reach USD 8.7 billion by 2023 from an estimated USD 6.0 billion in 2018, at a compound annual growth rate (CAGR) of 7.7% [20].

The production of typical strip assay includes the preparation of colloidal gold conjugates, application of reagents onto the membrane and pads, lamination of the strip membranes onto a support backing, cutting the prepared master cards into strips of defined length and width, and strip packaging (**Figure 1A** and **B**).

Three types of pads, a sample pad, conjugate pad, and absorbent pad, and nitrocellulose membrane are used for developing the strip assay. The test sample is applied onto the sample pad. Conjugate pad contains Abs, aptamers, or nucleic acids specific to the target analyte which are usually conjugated to colored particles, gold nanoparticles (GNPs), and latex beads. Capture reagents such as anti-target Abs or aptamers are immobilized in a line across the membrane which are nitrocellulose or cellulose acetate as a test line. It has also a control line containing capture reagents such as Abs or complementary nucleic acids specific for the conjugate Abs or aptamers present on the conjugate, respectively. The strip components are usually fixed to an inert backing material and may be placed in a plastic casing with a sample port, and reaction window showing the test and control line or strip can be prepared as a simple dipstick format [22]. After soaking of sample pad with analyte, it flows through the conjugate pad and nitrocellulose membrane via capillary action and ends on an absorbent pad. When the flow is continuing, the analyte bound by gold conjugate on conjugate pad is captured and accumulated on test line. The excess conjugate is also captured by a control line, and it should always be visible. If the test strip works correctly and it is positive, both the test and control lines are seen as red. If no colored capture lines or only a red color at the test line appears, the strip is invalid, and the test should be repeated [21, 23, 24] (**Figure 2**).

Although LFAs for *Salmonella* are commonly noncompetitive, the competitive format of LFA can also be developed for the smaller analytes [25, 26]. The principle of this

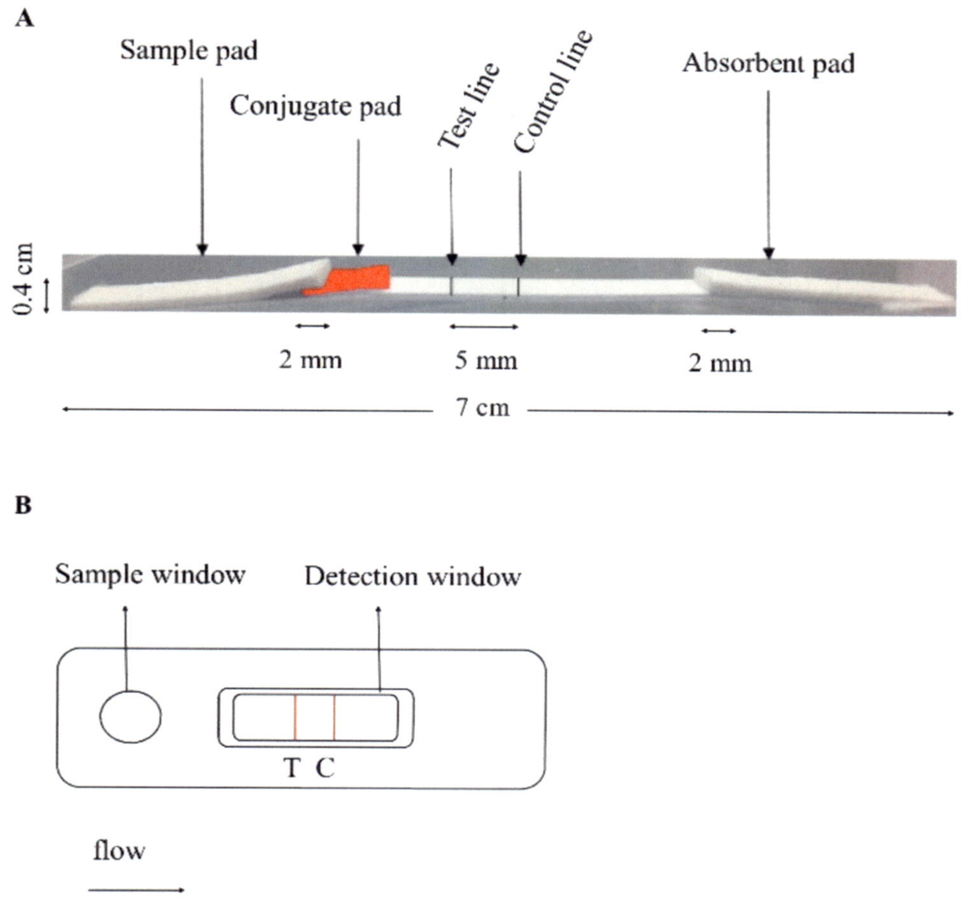

Figure 1.
Preparation of LFA strip (a) and schematic representation of it in plastic case [21].

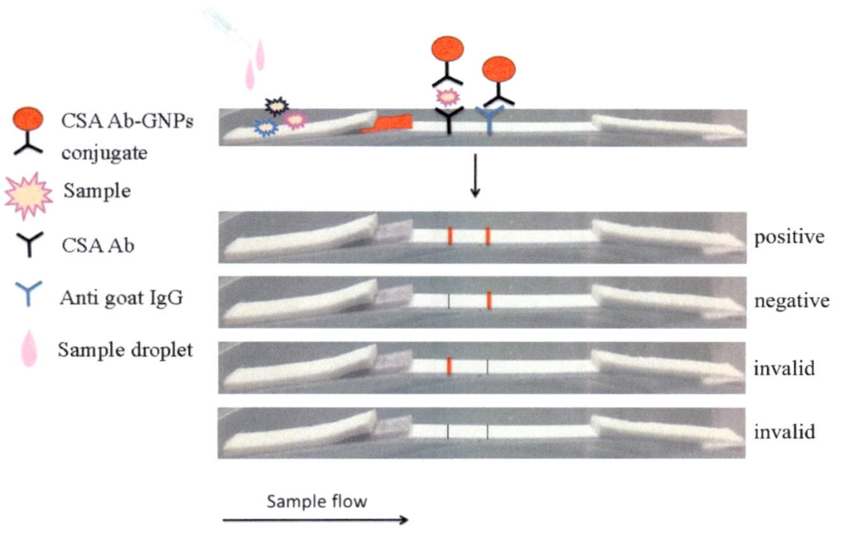

Figure 2.
Schematic diagram of the immunochromatographic test strip principle for the dipstick assay. CSA Ab, common structural antigenic antibody; GNPs, gold nanoparticles [21].

format is that sample extract is applied onto the sample pad and it flows through the absorbent pad. If the analyte is absent, all of the detection reagent would be trapped by capture reagent to form an easily visible test line. However, when the analyte is present, it competes with the immobilized capture reagent for the limited amount of competitive detection reagent. Thus, it means that the more analyte in the sample, the weaker the test line color.

Manufacturing of LFAs developed for *Salmonella* depends on some significant factors. First is the membrane type having suitable flow rate because it plays significant role for recognizing the whole bacteria cell. For instance, nitrocellulose Millipore membrane, Hi-Flow™ Plus 180 Membrane Card, shows good assay performance in terms of the whole-cell detection, analysis time, no background signal, and immobilization of capture reagents such as Abs and aptamers. If the flow rate of membrane is very slow, it takes a long time to see the results with the naked eye. However, if flow is very fast, capturing process cannot be completed and line intensities become unclear. Second is the application of analyte on sample pad. Both the dipstick assay and loading of sample as droplets can be preferred. The disadvantage of dipping the strip into bacterial media directly is that flow can be retarded on conjugate pad because of the media components. Thus, using the suitable running buffer, simple phosphate buffer saline (PBS), may enable conjugate to flow through the strip test, efficiently [21, 27]. Third is the immobilization of capture reagents. Generally streptavidin-biotin interaction is used for aptamer- or nucleic acid-based LFAs, and it sometimes may be required as multiple loading with consistent durations, while Abs can be directly immobilized once. The last one is the size of GNPs used for labeling. Although various studies showed that the size of GNPs between 15 and 40 nm can be used in LFAs, 35 nm GNPs are preferable. **Figure 3** displays the Ab-based LFAs for *Salmonella* when they are alone and present in bacterial mixture after optimal conditions are performed [27]. Strips were prepared by common structural Ab specific to *Salmonella enterica* species (*S. enteritidis*, *S. typhimurium*,

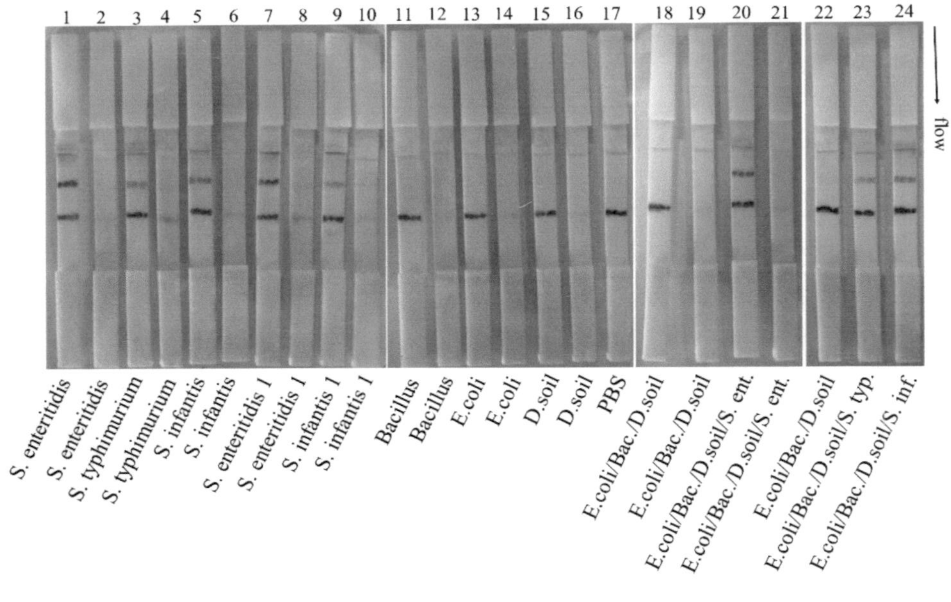

Figure 3.
Dipstick assay for live Salmonella *strains alone and in the mixture using M180 membrane. Test line:* Salmonella *Ab. Control line: Antigoat IgG. The strips were dipped into 200 μL of total bacteria with PBS. The strips 2–4–6–8–10–12–14–16–19–21 were prepared by naked GNPs. D. soil, dry soil bacteria; Bac,* B. cereus*; S. ent,* S. enteritidis*; S. typ,* S. typhimurium *[27].*

S. infantis). Bacteria isolated from the food samples were used. Dry soil bacteria, *E. coli*, *Bacillus*, and PBS were used as negative control. After culturing, test strips were dipped into the bacterial media without any treatment and showed positive results with target and nontarget samples. To highlight developed strip assays have high sensitivity and selectivity for the targets without non-specific interactions with the membrane and other samples.

The sensitivity and susceptibility of LFAs may also be improved by using high-affinity reagents including recombinant antibodies (Abs), one-step GNPs, or silver enhancement and integration of microfluidic papers with onboard electronics. Therefore, sensitive detection of *Salmonella* such as 10^2 or 102 cfu/mL is achieved for multiple recognition. Although cultural techniques associated with biochemical and serological confirmation tests and molecular methods are being developed for sensitive detection, they are time-consuming processes and not practical for end users. Thus, LFAs for *Salmonella* became attractive to make a rapid and sensitive detection for various species without nucleic acid isolation and advanced equipments. It is also open to improvement by integrating various detection systems for multiple recognition.

3. Antibodies for LFAs

Abs are more common reagents used for LFAs and available from a number of commercial sources. Various kinds of Abs generated by different ways includes recombinant protein technology, phage display technology, and hybridoma techniques. Although LFAs developed by monoclonal or polyclonal Ab are commonly in use, there are highly limited sources of LFA based on single-chain variable fragments (scFvs) [28]. Generally, commercial Abs used for sandwich assay in LFA might be obtained as prequalified by the vendor in pairs. These pairs are most readily available for relatively common and high-volume assays, such as tests for pregnancy, infectious disease, cardiac markers, and malignancies. Abs specific to various antigens of *Salmonella* species are in use for the development of LFAs [27, 29–31]. The common Ab-based LFAs for *Salmonella* recognition require these steps: (i) coating of GNPs with target specific Abs (detection Abs) via chemical or physical adsorption under the optimal pH value, (ii) immobilization of capture Abs on nitrocellulose membrane, and (iii) preparation of the pad and running buffers which has the optimal releasing effect through the membrane. The first use of Abs with colloidal gold reagent for a diagnostic immunoassay was reported in 1981 [32]. The optimal concentration of Abs to cover the GNPs and preventing them from agglomeration can be changeable. The specificity and selectivity of the strip assay depends on the affinity of used Abs. Thus, using high-affinity Abs will increase the sensitivity and decrease the limit of detection (LOD) and non-specific interactions with different antigens. To achieve this goal, engineered Abs are being continued to generate and adapt to LFAs, recently [33, 34]. As it is seen on **Figure 3**, all the requirements for LFAs mentioned above were achieved by Ab-based strip assay. Therefore, it makes possible to develop the strip assay for multiple *Salmonella* detection using both the monoclonal or polyclonal Abs on one assay.

4. Aptamers for LFAs

Aptamers are single-stranded DNA or RNA molecules that bind to the specific targets. Usage of aptamers in biosensors and development of new diagnostic systems based on aptamers become popular since 2000. Because they have high affinity to their targets, their generation is rapid and easy compared to the Abs, and conjugation with GNPs is chemical which is basically performed by thiol bonds. Besides, aptamer conjugates have long shelf life without degradation in comparison to Abs. Although they are used for developing LFAs, recently studies have still limited numbers in terms of the technical and application. While aptamers can be used together with Abs, they are commonly used as pairs for developing LFAs, and they should be decided carefully. Recognition aptamers present on GNPs and capture aptamers immobilized on the capture lines should have different binding sites to increase the sensitivity. Some LFAs for *Salmonella* detection based on aptamers are recorded in the literature with various reagents and techniques [35, 36]. While some aptamers show lower LOD such as 10^1 colony forming unit (cfu) of *S. enteritidis* [37], some of them show higher. Those variabilities can be caused by some reasons which are choosing the aptamer pairs, the distance of aptamers from the immobilization zone of membrane, affinity of aptamers [37, 38], and experimental assay conditions. Although large numbers of aptamers were recorded in the literature [39–41], there is still a lack of their adaptation to LFAs for the recognition of *Salmonella* species. Because the optimization of test parameters including immobilization procedure of aptamers on capture zones, optimal buffer ingredients, and membrane types, the exact size of GNPs has more complexity than Ab-based strip assays. Therefore, LFAs should be manufactured by high-affinity aptamers to detect whole *Salmonella* cells.

Nucleic acid-based LFAs using nucleic acid hybridization or amplification methods are also developed for *Salmonella*. However, further experimental steps including nucleic acid or genomic DNA isolation, primer design, and PCR are required. Due to the poorly suited point-of-care testing of PCR, new methods such as isothermal amplification become popular. The most common isothermal amplification methods are loop-mediated amplification (LAMP) [42, 43], nucleic acid sequence-based amplification (NASBA), rolling circle amplification (RCA), nicking enzyme-mediated amplification (NEMA), recombinase polymerase amplification (RPA), helicase-dependent amplification (HDA), multiple displacement amplification (MDA), and transcription-mediated amplification (TMA) depending on the detection techniques [44, 45]. Using this type of LFAs, lower detection limit of

	Detection	Detection reagent	Detection limit	Detection type	Refs.
S. typhimurium	LPS	Ab	-	Multiple	[29]
S. typhimurium	Whole cell	Ab	10^2 cfu/mL^{-1}	Single	[50]
Salmonella typhi	Whole cell	Ab	3×10^8 cfu	Single	[30]
S. typhimurium	16S ribosomal RNA and DNA	Nucleic acid-Ab	10^4 cells	Single	[51]
S. pullorum	Salmonella invA gene	Nucleic acid-Ab	89 fg/μl	Single	[52]
S. typhimurium	*Salmonella enterica* yfiR(375 bp) gene	Nucleic acid-Ab	0.75 pgμL^{-1}	Single	[49]
S. enteriditis	Out membrane of *S. enteritidis*	Aptamer	10 cfu mL^{-1}	Single	[37]
S. typhimurium	Whole cell	Aptamer	85 cfu mL^{-1}	Multiplex	[36]
S. typhimurium	Whole cell	Aptamer	-	Single	[35]

Table 1.
LFAs for Salmonella *detection by Ab, aptamer, and nucleic acids.*

Salmonella such as 20 fg of target DNA or 1.05×10^1 cfu of bacteria in pure culture [46] or 1.3–1.9 cfu/g or 1.3–1.9 cfu/mL of *Salmonella* in contaminated chicken products can be achieved after enrichment [47]. The assay sensitivity may also show variety according to the length of amplicon or target [48]. The commonly used reagents in this assay are biotin/fluorescein, biotin/digoxigenin tags for amplicons and gold/anti-digoxin Ab or gold/streptavidin conjugate on conjugate pad. Depending on the immobilized capture agents such as Abs, labeled nucleic acids, or aptamers on test and control line, assay is performed and results become visible for *Salmonella* [49]. **Table 1** shows some LFAs for *Salmonella* detection by using reagents mentioned above.

5. Gold nanoparticles for LFAs

Currently the nanoscale properties of GNPs have attracted more attention, and they are used in different fields like electronics [53], optics [54], and biosensors [55]. A common way to synthesize the nearly monodisperse spherical GNPs is the aqueous reduction of $HAuCl4$ by sodium citrate at boiling point [56]. Other reducing agents such as borohydrides and amines have also been used [57].

The nature of the surface chemistry of GNPs promotes easy and controlled attachment of other molecules especially those with thiol functionalities. Following their biocompatibility, high stability, ease of characterization [58, 59], and the controllable morphology, GNP-based bioconjugates are found to be good candidates for biomedical applications because they are stable with their conjugated parts compared to the unbound forms. If sodium chloride is present in the solution, repulsive and attractive forces between the particles are imbalanced, due to the masking of negative charge of colloidal solution [60]. This resulted with collapsing of gold particles after adsorbing one particle onto another, and visualization of this phenomenon is seen as the color change of colloids. However, in the presence of coating molecules including proteins, nucleic acids, and aptamers, they adsorb onto gold particles and help in preventing them from aggregation by inhibiting the binding of other gold particles. To make GNP conjugates, physical interaction is the simple method, while chemical interaction is also another method including covalent conjugation [61] by using thiol derivatives and bifunctional linkers.

LFAs based on GNPs conjugates have become useful innovation in nanotechnology. Colloidal gold is the most widely used label today in commercial LFAs for many reasons. It is fairly easy and inexpensive to prepare in the laboratory. The color is intense, and no development process is needed for visualization. However, assays may have varying sensitivity with respect to their target agents [22] in LFAs.

As a conclusion LFA based on GNPs is rapid and sensitive assay for *Salmonella* detection as point-of-care tests compared to other detection methods because it is a naked-eye analysis test and does not require the skilled personnel. Once it is developed, it can be used for 1 year by the end users without advanced equipments. Adapting different reagents including Abs, aptamers, or nucleic acids onto LFAs is another advantage because of their practical immobilization and binding steps in terms of the whole-cell detection and also their potential to be adopted to enhance LFAs.

Acknowledgements

The author acknowledges Prof. Dr. Hüseyin Avni ÖKTEM for advisory.

Conflict of interest

The author has read and approved the paper. The author agrees to the contents of the paper and has no conflict of interest.

Author details

Dilek ÇAM
Department of Biology, Faculty of Science, Çankırı Karatekin University, Çankırı, Turkey

*Address all correspondence to: cam.dilek@gmail.com

References

[1] Borch E, Nesbakken T, Christensen H. Hazard identification in swine slaughter with respect to foodborne bacteria. International Journal of Food Microbiology. 1996;**30**(1):9-25. DOI: 10.1016/0168-1605(96)00988-9

[2] Scientific Report of EFSA and ECDC. The European Union summary report on trends and sources of zoonoses, zoonotic agents and food-borne outbreaks in 2010. EFSA Journal. 2012;**10**(3):2597. DOI: 10.2903/j.efsa.2012.2597

[3] Stone GG, Oberst RD, Hays MP, McVey S, Galland JC, Curtiss R, et al. Detection of *Salmonella typhimurium* from rectal swabs of experimentally infected beagles by short cultivation and PCR-hybridization. Journal of Clinical Microbiology. 1995;**33**(5):1292-1295. PMID: 7615744

[4] Wen CY, Hu J, Zhang ZL, Tian ZQ, Ou GP, Liao YL, et al. One-step sensitive detection of *Salmonella typhimurium* by coupling magnetic capture and fluorescence identification with functional nanospheres. Analytical Chemistry. 2013;**85**(2):1223-1230. DOI: 10.1021/ac303204q

[5] Wang L, Li Y, Mustapha A. Rapid and simultaneous quantitation of *Escherichia coli* O157: H7, *Salmonella*, and *Shigella* in ground beef by multiplex real-time PCR and immunomagnetic separation. Journal of Food Protection. 2007;**70**(6):1366-1372. DOI: 10.4315/0362-028X-70.6.1366

[6] Woods DF, Reen FJ, Gilroy D, Buckley J, Frye JG, Boyd EF. Rapid multiplex PCR and real-time TaqMan PCR assays for detection of *Salmonella enterica* and the highly virulent serovars Choleraesuis and Paratyphi C. Journal of Clinical Microbiology. 2008;**46**(12):4018-4022. DOI: 10.1128/JCM.01229-08

[7] Kim S, Frye JG, Hu J, Fedorka-Cray PJ, Gautom R, Boyle DS. Multiplex PCR-based method for identification of common clinical serotypes of *Salmonella enterica* subsp. enterica. Journal of Clinical Microbiology. 2006;**44**(10):3608-3615. DOI: 10.1128/JCM.00701-06

[8] O'Regan E, McCabe E, Burgess C, McGuinness S, Barry T, Duffy G, et al. Development of a real-time multiplex PCR assay for the detection of multiple salmonella serotypes in chicken samples. BMC Microbiology. 2008;**8**(156):1-11. DOI: 10.1186/1471-2180-8-156

[9] Rajtak U, Leonard N, Bolton D, Fanning S. A real-time multiplex SYBR green I polymerase chain reaction assay for rapid screening of *Salmonella* serotypes prevalent in the European Union. Foodborne Pathogens and Disease. 2011;**8**(7):769-780. DOI: 10.1089/fpd.2010.0768

[10] Sapparapu G. Development of immunological reagents for detecting *Salmonella enterica* Serovar Typhimurium [thesis]. USA: University of Florida; 2003

[11] ZhangD, AlociljaEC. Characterization of nanoporous silicon-based DNA biosensor for the detection of *Salmonella enteritidis*. Sensors Journal, IEEE. 2008;**8**(6):775-780. DOI: 10.1109/JSEN.2008.923037

[12] Zuo P, Li X, Dominguez DC, Ye BC. A PDMS/paper/glass hybrid microfluidic biochip integrated with aptamer-functionalized graphene oxide nano-biosensors for one-step multiplexed pathogen detection. Lab on a Chip. 2013;**13**(19):3921-3928. DOI: 10.1039/c3lc50654a

[13] Kim G, Moon JH, Moh CY, Lim JG. A microfluidic nano-biosensor for the detection of pathogenic

salmonella. Biosensors and Bioelectronics. 2015;**67**:243-247. DOI: 10.1016/j.bios.2014.08.023

[14] Kohn J. An immunochromatographic technique. Immunology. 1968;**15**(6): 863-865. PMID: 4974484

[15] Laderman EI, Whitworth E, Dumaual E, Jones M, Hudak A, Hogrefe W, et al. Rapid, sensitive, and specific lateral-flow immunochromatographic point-of-care device for detection of herpes simplex virus type 2-specific immunoglobulin G antibodies in serum and whole blood. Clinical and Vaccine Immunology. 2008;**15**(1):159-163. DOI: 10.1128/CVI.00218-07

[16] He Y, Zhang S, Zhang X, Baloda M, Gurung AS, Xu H, et al. Ultrasensitive nucleic acid biosensor based on enzyme-gold nanoparticle dual label and lateral flow strip biosensor. Biosensors and Bioelectronics. 2011;**26**(5):2018-2024. DOI: 10.1016/j.bios.2010.08.079

[17] Ang GY, Yu CY, Yean CY. Ambient temperature detection of PCR amplicons with a novel sequence-specific nucleic acid lateral flow biosensor. Biosensors and Bioelectronics. 2012;**38**(1):151-156. DOI: 10.1016/j.bios.2012.05.019

[18] Ijeh M. Covalent gold nanoparticle—Antibody conjugates for sensitivity improvement in LFIA [thesis]. Germany: Hamburg University; 2011

[19] O'Farrell B. Evolution in lateral flow-based immunoassay systems. In: Wong R, Tse H, editors. Lateral Flow Immunoassay. USA: Humana Press; 2009. pp. 1-33. DOI: 10.1007/978-1-59745-240-3_1

[20] Lateral Flow Assay Market by Application (Clinical Testing (Pregnancy, Infectious Disease (Mosquito , Influenza, STI, Hepatitis, TB), Cardiac Marker, Lipid Test) Veterinary, Food Safety) Product (Reader, Kits) Technique, End User—Global Forecast to 2023 [Internet]. 2017. Available from: https://www.marketsandmarkets.com/Market-Reports/lateral-flow-assay-market-167205133.html

[21] Çam D, Öktem HA. Optimizations needed for lateral flow assay for rapid detection of pathogenic *E. coli*. Turkish Journal of Biology. 2017;**41**:954-968. DOI: 10.3906/biy-1705-50

[22] Peruski AH, Peruski LF. Immunological methods for detection and identification of infectious disease and biological warfare agents. Clinical and Diagnostic Laboratory Immunology. 2003;**10**(4):506-513. DOI: 10.1128/CDLI.10.4.506-513.2003

[23] Song C, Liu Q, Zhi A, Yang J, Zhi Y, Li Q, et al. Development of a lateral flow colloidal gold immunoassay strip for the rapid detection of olaquindox residues. Journal of Agricultural and Food Chemistry. 2011;**59**(17):9319-9326. DOI: 10.1021/jf202213m

[24] Tripathi V, Nara S, Singh K, Singh H, Shrivastav TG. A competitive immunochromatographic strip assay for 17-α-hydroxy progesterone using colloidal gold nanoparticles. Clinica Chimica Acta. 2012;**413**(1):262-268. DOI: 10.1016/j.cca.2011.10.016

[25] Zhang GP, Wang XN, Yang JF, Yang YY, Xing GX, Li QM, et al.Development of an immunochromatographic lateral flow test strip for detection of β-adrenergic agonist clenbuterol residues. Journal of Immunological Methods. 2006;**312**(1):27-33. DOI: 10.1016/j.jim.2006.02.017

[26] Molinelli A, Grossalber K, Krska R. A rapid lateral flow test for the determination of total type B fumonisins in maize. Analytical and Bioanalytical Chemistry.

2009;**395**(5):1309-1316. DOI: 0.1007/s00216-009-3082-4

[27] Çam D, Öktem HA. Development of rapid dipstick assay for food pathogens, *Salmonella*, by optimized parameters. Journal of Food Science and Technology. 2019;**56**(1):140-148. DOI: 10.1007/s13197-018-3467-5

[28] Wemmer S, Mashau C, Fehrsen J, Van Wyngaardt W, Du Plessis DH. Chicken scFvs and bivalent scFv-C H fusions directed against HSP65 of *Mycobacterium bovis*. Biologicals. 2010;**38**(3):407-414. DOI: 10.1016/j.biologicals.2010.02.002

[29] Schenk F, Weber P, Vogler J, Hecht L, Dietzel A, Gauglitz G. Development of a paper-based lateral flow immunoassay for simultaneous detection of lipopolysaccharides of *Salmonella* serovars. Analytical and Bioanalytical Chemistry. 2018;**410**:863-868. DOI: 10.1007/s00216-017-0643-9

[30] Lukman YM, Dyana ZN, Rahmah N, Khairunisak AR. Development and evaluation of colloidal gold lateral flow immunoassays for detection of *Escherichia Coli* O157 and *Salmonella Typhi*. IOP Conference Series: Journal of Physics: Conference Series. 2018;**1082**:012049. DOI: 10.1088/1742-6596/1082/1/012049

[31] Zhao Y, Wang H, Zhang P, Sun C, Wang X, Wang X, et al. Rapid multiplex detection of 10 foodborne pathogens with an up-converting phosphor technology-based 10-channel lateral flow assay. Scientific Reports. 2016;**6**:1-8. DOI: 10.1038/srep21342

[32] Leuvering JH, Thal PJ, Van der Waart M, Schuurs AH. A sol particle agglutination assay for human chorionic gonadotrophin. Journal of Immunological Methods. 1981;**45**(2):183-194. DOI: 10.1016/0022-1759(81)90212-X

[33] Melnik S, Neumann AC, Karongo R, Dirndorfer S, Stübler M, Ibl V, et al. Cloning and plant-based production of antibody MC10E7 for a lateral flow immunoassay to detect [4-arginine] microcystin in freshwater. Plant Biotechnology Journal. 2018;**16**(1):27-38. DOI: 10.1111/pbi.12746

[34] Gandhi S, Banga I, Maurya PK, Eremin SA. A gold nanoparticle-single-chain fragment variable antibody as an immunoprobe for rapid detection of morphine by dipstick. RSC Advances. 2018;**8**(3):1511-1518. DOI: 10.1039/c7ra12810j

[35] Bruno JG. Application of DNA aptamers and quantum dots to lateral flow test strips for detection of foodborne pathogens with improved sensitivity versus colloidal gold. Pathogens. 2014;**3**(2):341-355. DOI: 10.3390/pathogens3020341

[36] Jin B, Yang Y, He R, Park YI, Leee A, Bai D, et al. Lateral flow aptamer assay integrated smartphone-based portable device for simultaneous detection of multiple targets using upconversion nanoparticles. Sensors and Actuators B: Chemical. 2018;**276**:48-56. DOI: 10.1016/j.snb.2018.08.074

[37] Fang Z, Wu W, Lu X, Zeng L. Lateral flow biosensor for DNA extraction-free detection of *Salmonella* based on aptamer mediated strand displacement amplification. Biosensors and Bioelectronics. 2014;**56**:192-197. DOI: 10.1016/j.bios.2014.01.015

[38] Park HC, Baig IA, Lee SC, Moon JY, Yoon MY. Development of ssDNA aptamers for the sensitive detection of *Salmonella typhimurium* and *Salmonella enteritidis*. Applied Biochemistry and Biotechnology. 2014;**174**(2):793-802. DOI: 10.1007/s12010-014-1103-z

[39] Book B, Chen J, Irudayaraj J. Quantification of receptor targeting aptamer binding characteristics

using single-molecule spectroscopy. Biotechnology and Bioengineering. 2011;**108**(5):1222-1227. DOI: 10.1002/bit.23043

[40] Duan N, Wu S, Chen X, Huang Y, Xia Y, Ma X, et al. Selection and characterization of aptamers against *Salmonella typhimurium* using whole-bacterium systemic evolution of ligands by exponential enrichment (SELEX). Journal of Agricultural and Food Chemistry. 2013;**61**(13):3229-3234. DOI: 10.1021/jf400767d

[41] Ning Y, Li W, Duan Y, Yang M, Deng L. High specific DNAzyme-aptamer sensor for *Salmonella paratyphi* a using single-walled nanotubes-based dual fluorescence-spectrophotometric methods. Journal of Biomolecular Screening. 2014;**19**(7):1099-1106. DOI: 10.1177/1087057114528538

[42] Perera RS, Ding XC, Tully F, Oliver J, Bright N, et al. Development and clinical performance of high throughput loop-mediated isothermal amplification for detection of malaria. PLoS One. 2017;**12**(2):e0171126. DOI: 10.1371/journal.pone.0171126

[43] Kokkinos PA, Ziros PG, Bellou M, Vantarakis A. Loop-mediated isothermal amplification (LAMP) for the detection of *Salmonella* in food. Food Analytical Methods. 2014;**7**(2):512-526. DOI: 10.1007/s12161-013-9748-8

[44] Kaur A, Kapil A, Elangovan R, Jha S, Kalyanasundaram D. Highly sensitive detection of *Salmonella typhi* in clinical blood samples by magnetic nanoparticle-based enrichment and in-situ measurement of isothermal amplification of nucleic acids. PLoS One. 2018;**13**(3):e0194817. DOI: 10.1371/journal.pone.0194817

[45] Zanoli L, Spoto G. Isothermal amplification methods for the detection of nucleic acids in microfluidic devices. Biosensors. 2013;**3**(1):18-43. DOI: 10.3390/bios3010018

[46] Liu H, Zang YX, Du XJ, Li P, Wang S. Development of an isothermal amplification-based assay for the rapid visual detection of salmonella bacteria. Journal of Dairy Science. 2017;**100**(9):7016-7025. DOI: 10.3168/jds.2017-12566

[47] Du XJ, Zhou TJ, Li P, Wang S. A rapid salmonella detection method involving thermophilic helicase-dependent amplification and a lateral flow assay. Molecular and Cellular Probes. 2017;**34**:37-44. DOI: 10.1016/j.mcp.2017.05.004

[48] Bulut O. Development of nucleic acid based lateral flow immunochromatographic test platform for *Salmonella* detection [thesis]. Turkey: Middle East Technical University; 2014

[49] Aissa AB, Jara JJ, Sebastián RM, Vallribera A, Campoy S, Pividori MI. Comparing nucleic acid lateral flow and electrochemical genosensing for the simultaneous detection of foodborne pathogens. Biosensors and Bioelectronics. 2017;**88**:265-272. DOI: 10.1016/j.bios.2016.08.046

[50] Park TS, Li W, McCracken KE, Yoon JY. Smartphone quantifies *Salmonella* from paper microfluidics. Lab on a Chip. 2013;**13**(24):4832-4840. DOI: 10.1039/c3lc50976a

[51] Liu CC, Yeung CY, Chen PH, Yeh MK, Hou SY. Salmonella detection using 16S ribosomal DNA/RNA probe-gold nanoparticles and lateral flow immunoassay. Food Chemistry. 2013;**141**:2526-2532. DOI: 10.1016/j.foodchem.2013.05.089

[52] Liu ZK, Zhang QY, Yang NN, Xu MG, Xu JF, Jing ML, et al. Rapid and sensitive detection of salmonella in chickens using loop-mediated isothermal amplification combined

with a lateral flow dipstick. Journal of Microbiology and Biotechnology. 2019;**29**(3):454-464. DOI: 10.4014/jmb.1712.12010

[53] Rothenberg E, Kazes M, Shaviv E, Banin U. Electric field induced switching of the fluorescence of single semiconductor quantum rods. Nano Letters. 2005;**5**(8):1581-1586. DOI: 10.1021/nl051007n

[54] Yao JL, Pan GP, Xue KH, Wu DY, Ren B, Sun DM, et al. A complementary study of surface-enhanced Raman scattering and metal nanorod arrays. Pure and Applied Chemistry. 2000;**72**(1):221-228. DOI: 10.1351/pac200072010221

[55] Aslan K, Zhang J, Lakowicz JR, Geddes CD. Saccharide sensing using gold and silver nanoparticles-a review. Journal of Fluorescence. 2004;**14**(4):391-400. DOI: 10.1023/B:JOFL.0000031820.17358.28

[56] Narayanan R, El-Sayed MA. Catalysis with transition metal nanoparticles in colloidal solution: Nanoparticle shape dependence and stability. The Journal of Physical Chemistry B. 2005;**109**(26):12663-12676. DOI: 10.1021/jp051066p

[57] Wilson OM, Hu X, Cahill DG, Braun PV. Colloidal metal particles as probes of nanoscale thermal transport in fluids. Physical Review B. 2002;**66**(22):224301. DOI: 10.1103/PhysRevB.66.224301

[58] Nie S, Emory SR. Probing single molecules and single nanoparticles by surface-enhanced Raman scattering. Science. 1997;**275**(5303):1102-1106. DOI: 10.1126/science.275.5303.1102

[59] Sperling RA, Gil PR, Zhang F, ZanellaM,ParakWJ.Biologicalapplications of gold nanoparticles. Chemical Society Reviews. 2008;**37**(9):1896-1908. DOI: 10.1039/b712170a

[60] Derjaguin BV, Landau L. Theory of the stability of strongly charged lyophobic sols and of the adhesion of strongly charged particles in solutions of electrolytes. Acta Physicochim URSS. 1941;**14**(6):633-662. NAID: 10016600848

[61] Caruso F. Nanoengineering of particle surfaces. Advanced Materials. 2001;**13**(1):11-22. DOI: 10.1002/1521-4095(200101)13:1<11:AID-ADMA11>3.0.CO;2-N

Chapter 10

Applications of Genomics in Regulatory Food Safety Testing in Canada

Catherine D. Carrillo, Adam Koziol, Neil Vary and Burton W. Blais

Abstract

Recent developments in the field of pathogen genomics herald a new paradigm for analytical food microbiology in which pathogenic bacteria will be characterized on the basis of their genetic profile rather than traditional approaches relying on phenotypic properties. The ability to identify gene markers associated with virulence, antimicrobial resistance, and other properties relevant to the identification, risk profiling, and typing of foodborne bacterial isolates will play a critical role in informing regulatory decisions and tracing sources of food contamination. Here we present several scenarios illustrating current and prospective roles for pathogen genomics in food inspection.

Keywords: pathogen genomics, virulence, foodborne pathogens, whole-genome sequencing, typing, bioinformatics, food inspection, *Escherichia coli*, *Salmonella*, *Listeria*

1. Introduction

The food microbiology testing laboratory has a key role in supporting regulatory food safety investigations, whether stemming from a contamination incident identified through routine monitoring food inspection programs or a foodborne illness outbreak event where human lives and well-being are at risk. While such investigations typically involve the concerted actions of food inspection and public health authorities at different levels of government, the main role of the regulatory testing laboratory is to confirm the presence of a specified hazard in a food vehicle and provide data indicating the scope and source of a contamination event. The extent to which the laboratory can contribute critical information to an investigation will to a large degree depend on the application of leading-edge technologies for detection and characterization of foodborne pathogens. Approaches capable of maximizing the amount of information obtained in the course of conducting laboratory testing of inspection samples will foster the most appropriate regulatory responses, for example, by informing the health risk assessment process undertaken to categorize the degree of risk attending a contamination incident.

The impact of analytical service delivery on public health outcomes depends on the ability to process large numbers of investigative samples and produce accurate test results in the shortest timeframe possible. While cultural enrichment of food samples to amplify pathogens to detectable levels is generally necessary for their recovery, current approaches often use protracted identification processes relying on phenotypic characteristics elucidated by time-consuming cultivation, biochemical and serological techniques. While effective under certain circumstances, there are shortcomings to such a limited approach, when dealing with novel pathogens for which analytical parameters may not have been comprehensively worked out or in trying to attribute contamination sources.

The exploitation of the genetic blueprint, or known parts thereof, associated with a targeted bacterial pathogen is now widely accepted as an effective means for the identification of food pathogens. Polymerase chain reaction (PCR) technology is now well established as an analytical tool in the regulatory food laboratory [1–4]. Its implementation in regulatory testing programs underscores the growing acceptance of redefining the terms for the identification and characterization of bacteria from a phenotypic to a genotypic basis. Indeed, the advent of leading-edge genomics technologies opens new possibilities for comprehensive analyses of microbial isolates recovered from food inspection samples; for example, next-generation sequencing technologies (whole-genome sequencing, WGS) can now render a bacterial genome much faster (i.e., within 1–3 days) and at a significantly lower cost (about 100 dollars) than previously possible, making it feasible to sequence foodborne isolates within the timeframes of food safety investigations [5–7].

Currently available bioinformatics tools are sufficiently advanced to enable the rapid processing of raw sequence data into a usable form for many purposes. Sequencing pathogenic bacteria, whether in the context of outbreak investigations or information gathering in the course of research, can yield an unprecedented level of information regarding the presence of virulence and other marker genes relevant to the identification and risk characterization of food isolates [6–10]. WGS data can provide an exquisite degree of resolution capable of ascertaining differences between strains and determining phylogenetic relationships among different bacterial isolates for pinpoint precision in the attribution of contamination sources [6, 11]. Finally, the identification of strain-specific features such as unique DNA sequences, metabolic properties, and antimicrobial resistance will enable testing labs to implement customized tests addressing specific strains of interest in determining the scope of contamination events.

While genomics, including WGS technology, already plays a significant role in the clinical sciences, its role in regulatory food microbiology inspection programs remains to be fully delineated. Currently, methods used to characterize foodborne pathogens recovered in regulatory food testing programs aim to answer three questions: (1) what is it? (2) have we seen it before? and (3) is it dangerous? This work describes some of the ways in which characterization of bacterial pathogens using genomics technologies has provided or may contribute to faster, more reliable and cost-effective results addressing these questions. Our purpose is to present different scenarios to illustrate impacts of leading-edge genomics technologies, some imagined, and others already achieved, on food inspection programs.

2. Impacts of the implementation of genomics in regulatory food microbiology

2.1 What is it? Definitive identification of pathogenic bacteria based on genomics techniques

2.1.1 In the beginning: detection of genomic markers by PCR

Escherichia coli O157:H7 have been implicated in outbreaks of foodborne illness associated with the consumption of contaminated foods such as ground beef and produce [12, 13]. In the event of an outbreak, it is imperative that production lots associated with the primary food vehicle are identified as quickly as possible in order to recall all contaminated products from the marketplace [14]. Traditional techniques for the detection of *E. coli* O157:H7 in foods rely on a multistep process involving pre-enrichment in a selective broth followed by plating to reveal the presence of sorbitol-negative colonies, which are then purified and subjected to a battery of biochemical and serological tests to confirm their identity [15, 16]. This process can take up to 1 week to complete before the contaminant can be definitively identified because of the requirement for growth and phenotypic expression of the organism.

As an alternative to classic phenotypic techniques, the identification of foodborne colony isolates can be achieved on the basis of detection of defining gene markers. Detection platforms incorporating PCR techniques are particularly well suited for same-day analysis of a primary colony isolate. The CFIA microbiology laboratory network has undertaken a program of method development aimed at the rapid identification of colonies isolated on plating media at an early stage during the enrichment process. A key technology platform adopted by CFIA for this purpose is the cloth-based hybridization array system (CHAS) providing for identification of pathogens through amplification of key target genes by multiplex PCR, followed by rapid hybridization of the amplicons with an array of immobilized capture probes on a polyester cloth support [2–4, 17]. This approach enables facile detection of many gene markers in a single reaction, with specificity assured through the hybridization process.

A CHAS method for the identification of *E. coli* O157:H7 [17] has been validated following the guidelines of the Health Canada *Compendium of Analytical Methods* (CAM) (available at [18]). This method has been published in the CAM (MFLP-22: Characterization of verotoxigenic *Escherichia coli* O157:H7 colonies by polymerase chain reaction and cloth-based hybridization array system, [2]), enabling its implementation for regulatory testing purposes in Canada. It is notable as the first instance of a genetic marker-based approach for the definitive identification of a foodborne pathogen isolate in our laboratories. The *E. coli* O157:H7 CHAS was used by CFIA laboratories on two separate occasions in 2013 to provide critical evidence supporting health risk assessments in connection with foodborne illness outbreaks implicating ground beef distributed in Canada. This method enabled the testing laboratories to issue official results of analysis a full 2 days ahead of the traditional approach, leading to more timely interventions minimizing public exposure to the contaminated product. The CHAS technology has now been incorporated into routine diagnostic testing schemes in CFIA food testing laboratories.

2.1.2 Enter the next generation: whole-genome sequencing

Non-O157 STEC, particularly strains bearing certain O antigenic determinants (O26, O45, O103, O111, O121, O145, and O157), are emerging as a serious foodborne public health concern [19]. Unlike *E. coli* O157:H7, there are no biochemical features by which these so-called priority STEC strains can be differentiated from commensal *E. coli* or other STEC which are not a public health concern. However, it is universally recognized that foodborne STEC posing a public health risk can be defined on the basis of possession of certain gene markers, including the Shiga toxin genes *st1* or *st2*, the intimin-coding gene *eae*, and markers for the specific serogroups of concern [1, 19, 20]. Thus, priority STEC constitute a striking example illustrating the benefit of the use of gene markers for pinpointing pathogens otherwise not readily amenable to identification by classic means. This in turn has enabled practical strategies for multiplex gene detection methods for detection of such pathogens during routine monitoring of the food supply to verify industry compliance with food safety regulations. In fact, such an approach is the basis for the Canadian STEC Method which was developed jointly by CFIA and Health Canada for the detection of this family of pathogens in meats and produce [3, 4].

The potential of PCR technology to provide informative test results is limited by its rather fragmentary nature, that is, the fact that only a relatively small number of different DNA markers can be assessed in a single analytical procedure. A considerable effort is required to optimize and validate the performance of PCR systems, particularly those in which multiple primer pairs are combined (e.g., identification of priority Shiga toxigenic *E. coli* (STEC) using a combination of 11 primer pairs; [1]). For all intents and purposes, validated assays are locked into their original configurations, and it is not possible to modify them (e.g., add or alter primers) on an ad hoc basis without first having to undertake a laborious and time-consuming re-evaluation of assay performance characteristics. Thus, novel queries cannot be undertaken if, in the course of an active food safety investigation, new questions arise regarding the occurrence of an unanticipated assay target. This was the case in a 2011 German outbreak involving STEC with an unusual virulence profile [21, 22].

The use of WGS technologies for STEC characterization can provide a more complete picture [8]; however, completion of WGS analyses typically requires 3–5 days. As this timeline may be too long in an outbreak situation, we have developed practical processes in which genomic DNA isolated from a single STEC colony is sequenced using the Illumina MiSeq platform, followed by analysis of the sequence data during the course of the sequencing run for the determination of genomic markers for phylogenetic identity, virulence profile, serotyping, as well as biological metrics serving as quality control features supporting the validity of the process [5]. Identification and characterization of isolates can be completed within 9 h, comparable to the current method used for characterization of STEC. This real-time WGS approach produces high-resolution characterization of bacterial pathogens at a cost and within a timeframe that are similar to standard microbiological techniques and has the potential to replace lengthy biochemical characterization and molecular and serological typing procedures widely used in food testing laboratories. Our laboratory is currently studying strategies for broad implementation of WGS technology in support of regulatory food inspection objectives through the detection, identification, and characterization of priority bacterial pathogens such as STEC, *Salmonella enterica*, and *Listeria monocytogenes* [5, 23–25]. We have developed guidelines and implemented validated methods and bioinformatics tools for automated analyses of sequence data to ensure reliability and reproducibility of WGS-based analyses [24, 26].

2.2 Have we seen it before? Impact of high-resolution molecular typing by WGS for distinguishing new isolates from control and historical laboratory isolates

Following detection of a pathogen in foods, (sub)typing methods are often used to generate a profile of the isolated organism to determine similarity to previously characterized isolates from clinical or food sources (reviewed in [27–29]). Typing of isolates recovered from food samples can provide important information regarding the complexity and source(s) of a given contamination incident, enables tracking of foodborne bacterial strains, and is frequently used to support regulatory decisions.

Early methods of typing were based on phenotypic properties, for example, serotyping based on proteins expressed by the organism on surface structures [30–32] and phage typing based on susceptibility to reference panels of bacteriophage for distinguishing closely related isolates [33]. The development of methods based on DNA sequences followed [29]. Methods such as multilocus sequence typing

(MLST), involving sequencing of PCR-amplified fragments of a small number (i.e., 6–9) of housekeeping genes, can be used to infer evolutionary relationships among organisms [34, 35]. This portable and highly reproducible method of typing has been widely deployed, and MLST schema have been developed for all of the priority foodborne pathogens [34]. For public health surveillance in Canada, as in other jurisdictions, the standard approach for typing of foodborne pathogens for cluster identification has been pulsed-field gel electrophoresis (PFGE) and multilocus variable-number tandem repeat analysis (MLVA) [27, 28, 36, 37]. In North America, data is shared among public health agencies through PulseNet [27, 38]. The selection of a typing method depends on a number of factors, including proven utility of the method for the pathogen being investigated. Each method requires costly training of lab personnel and in many cases the purchase of specialized equipment [39]. Furthermore, comparisons of typing data among different strains can only be done in cases where the same method has been applied. In some cases, variability in the execution of methods by different analysts or different labs significantly impacts the comparability of molecular typing data [36].

These typing methods are based on a limited subset of genomic sequences and often lack the discriminatory power to differentiate among closely related organisms [39]. DNA typing profiles from two isolates appearing indistinguishable might be interpreted as evidence that the bacteria have a common source. However, the strength of this type of evidence rests on the extent to which the DNA profile consists of a combination of rare traits. When the traits defining a DNA profile are not rare, there is the possibility that two isolates are in fact unrelated and that matches are mere chance occurrences. In highly clonal strains (e.g., *Salmonella*) serovar Enteritidis, where only a few single-nucleotide changes may be observed among epidemiologically unrelated strains, most methods are not sufficiently discriminatory [40].

WGS provides a high-resolution molecular typing platform that can be universally applied to bacterial pathogens [6, 38, 41]. In principle, strains differing by even a single nucleotide can be distinguished [42, 43]. Furthermore, WGS can now be done more cheaply than lower resolution methods such as MLST and is backward-compatible with previous methods since, in some cases, typing data can be generated from minimally processed genomic data in silico [8, 9, 44]. Strains characterized by WGS can be compared to strains characterized by any other DNA-based subtyping method, enabling optimal use of historical data. Molecular typing data have generally been developed as a surrogate measure of the genetic similarity between bacterial strains. Using databases of WGS information, the utility of existing subtyping methods can be rigorously assessed, and improved subtyping schemes that reflect true strain relationships can be developed [45].

One advantage of the availability of WGS for typing bacterial isolates is the ability to evaluate datasets at different levels of resolution as needed to resolve biological questions. In this regard, MLST continues to be a valuable approach for tracking foodborne pathogens in the genomic era [41, 44]. WGS data can be matched to current and historical databases at different levels of resolution including pathogen-specific MLST (described above), core genome MLST (cgMLST) which uses hundreds of genes that are conserved within a species, and whole-genome MLST (wgMLST) which considers all genes within a species [38]. Similarly, ribosomal MLST (rMLST) is a 53-gene scheme with the advantage of being universally applicable to bacteria typically encountered in a food testing laboratory [46].

The highest-resolution WGS-based analyses such as wgMLST and single-nucleotide variant (SNV) analyses provide unrivaled DNA fingerprinting capability and offer tremendous potential for food safety applications [41, 42, 47]. Still, the use of these analyses in a food safety context is in its infancy, and the interpretation of genomic data from foodborne pathogens in support of regulatory interventions remains challenging [48]. For example, how many SNVs are required to exclude a sample from a food safety investigation? This question remains difficult to answer, in part because of differences in rates at which DNA accumulates changes within a species or among strains within a species. Bacterial strains with a mutator phenotype have an elevated mutation rate, typically due to mutations in genes encoding components of DNA replication and repair pathways [49]. Mutator phenotypes are commonly found in clinical bacterial populations and may contribute significantly to the acquisition of antimicrobial resistance [50–52]. For example, the mutator phenotype has been attributed to the development of multidrug-resistant *S. typhimurium* [50]. In *E. coli*, this phenotype has recently been shown to be induced in response to stress conditions [53]. The possibility that environmental stress could lead to the development of the mutator phenotype may be highly relevant to analyses of foodborne pathogens.

2.2.1 Identification of persistent contamination

Persistent contamination of food manufacturing environments with bacteria such as *Listeria monocytogenes* poses significant public health risks as these events serve as a source for the continual contamination of food products, primarily because (by definition) persistent contaminators defy attempts to sanitize the manufacturing environment using standard protocols [54–56]. *Listeria monocytogenes* is the causative agent of listeriosis, a potentially fatal foodborne illness in susceptible populations such as the very young, the elderly, and the immunocompromised [57]. The ability of this organism to contaminate food contact surfaces (e.g., conveyors, saws, etc.) and survive in the manufacturing environment increases the risk of food product contamination, with possible serious public health consequences. Routinely monitoring the food manufacturing environment for the presence of pathogenic bacteria is a key to preventing contamination of food products [56]. The presence of environmental contamination is usually ascertained through swabbing and testing of food manufacturing environment surfaces using standard microbiology techniques. Transient contamination is of a sporadic nature and may be effectively managed through the application of standard sanitation regimens followed by testing to ensure treatment efficacy. Persistent contamination occurs when a specific strain becomes a permanent resident of specific niches in the manufacturing environment. Persistence may be attributable to the incorporation of *L. monocytogenes* into biofilms occurring on equipment surfaces, resistance to commonly used sanitizers such as benzalkonium chloride, or through mechanical sequestration in hard-to-clean areas (e.g., meat cutting saw arbors, as was the case in the 2008 Canadian listeriosis outbreak resulting in many fatalities associated with the consumption of contaminated ready-to-eat meats [58]).

The ability to distinguish the two modes of contamination in the analysis of environmental isolates recovered during routine monitoring activities would constitute an important element to inform the best approach for the management of microbial hazards in food manufacturing plants [54, 55]. For example, while regular sanitation procedures may be effective in dealing with removal of sporadic surface contaminants, a more comprehensive approach requiring equipment teardown and aggressive sanitation would be required to deal with persistent contaminants, which are by nature highly resistant to sanitizers and cleaning procedures. The traditional approach to identify the occurrence of persistent contamination in food manufacturing environments involves the characterization of successive isolates using typing procedures such as PFGE to determine their relatedness [54]. However, PFGE is of limited value for this purpose because it is not sufficiently discriminatory to unequivocally establish whether two strains are clonally related (i.e., one being descendant from the other). Depending on the scope of the contamination, there may be multiple related populations within the food production environment.

Whole-genome sequencing approaches offer the prospect of determining the degree of relatedness among isolates on the basis of very fine base sequence differences, because more closely or clonally related isolates have fewer SNV differences. Therefore, it should be possible to compare two isolates (e.g., recovered on successive sampling incursions in the same plant) using high-resolution WGS typing methods to ascertain whether they are clonally related or different [55]. In the former case, this would be a strong indication that there is either an unresolved source of contamination in the plant, or more likely, a case of persistent contamination, whereas the latter case would suggest two independent contamination incidents. Each scenario would warrant a different approach to decontamination, and the ability to differentiate persistent and sporadic strains on the basis of the relatedness of successive isolates would constitute a powerful risk assessment and risk management tool for the use in the most highly proactive food safety programs. There is one caveat in the use of SNV-based typing, and that is the temporal drift which naturally occurs in bacteria, resulting in the accumulation of SNVs among the progeny derived from a single parent. The question remains under which conditions this occurs for bacterial strains in a food manufacturing environment and how many SNV differences constitute a real difference in terms of the provenance of isolates under comparison.

One cause of *L. monocytogenes* persistence has been identified as resistance to sanitizers such as quaternary ammonium compounds (QACs) [59–61]. An important determinant of QAC resistance is efflux systems such as those encoded by the *bcrABC* gene cassette [62] or *emrE* [63]. In a recent study to characterize the genomes of *L. monocytogenes* isolates collected at a pig slaughterhouse to determine the molecular basis for their persistence, we found that successive environmental isolates (persistent types) linked on the basis of SNV analyses all harbored the *bcrABC* and concluded that high-resolution typing and determination of the cassette may serve to distinguish between persistent and sporadic *L. monocytogenes* isolates [59]. This in turn may have important ramifications for risk management actions when *L. monocytogenes* is recovered from a food manufacturing environment, since the ability of a strain to persist casts doubt on the efficacy of standard sanitization protocols, and more intensive cleaning procedures (e.g., equipment teardown, use of alternative sanitizers) may be warranted. These types of analyses of food inspection isolates are greatly facilitated by WGS technology [55, 59].

2.2.2 Contribution to surveillance programs and outbreak investigations

Although numerous methods are used by food safety and public health agencies to support regulatory decisions during outbreak investigations, demonstrating that food and clinical isolates originated from the same source can be challenging. As the results generated by WGS make their way into situation rooms to guide decision-makers, concise metrics for the interpretation and contextualization of genomics-derived data will be required to achieve more precise assessments [64]. The value of WGS-based typing for cluster identification has already been demonstrated through global surveillance networks such as GenomeTrakr and PulseNet [6, 38, 41]. Smaller clusters of cases can be linked through WGS analyses and investigated [65], and conversely, unrelated cases can be excluded from an epidemiological investigation leading to improved outcomes for rapid identification of foods implicated in outbreaks [66]. Nonetheless, WGS results should not be interpreted in the absence of epidemiological context as some lineage rates of mutation are low and strains from different sources may appear to be linked [67].

The concepts of "match probability" and "likelihood ratios" are well known in human forensic sciences where they facilitate the interpretation of DNA profiles in matching individuals to a crime scene [68]. For example, when the DNA profile found on a crime scene matches that of a suspect and there is only a one-in-one million probability that this DNA profile might be found in another individual, there is a strong case linking the suspect to the crime scene. Food inspectors face a similar situation during outbreak investigations when trying to establish causal links between isolates from different sources [69]. Bacteria may undergo subtle changes in their genomes during the course of a foodborne illness outbreak event, with possible impacts on the typing profiles of clonally related isolates recovered over time. The question arises as to how much change in a genome constitutes a significant difference between individual isolates (i.e., different origins or strains). Through statistical analyses of comprehensive pathogen genome databases, it should be possible to develop a likelihood ratio approach to determine the probability of finding a given profile in a defined population and, hence, develop criteria to measure sequence diversity between isolates with different degrees of relatedness and even among clonally related isolates recovered over the course of an outbreak event [69]. This in turn would provide a greater degree of confidence in attributing the origins of isolates, identifying clusters of foodborne illness and their food vehicles, and the scope of contamination. This information can also be used to revise and adjust detection tools (e.g., PCR primers) to ensure their effectiveness in identifying "moving" genomic targets. The development of a forensic likelihood ratio approach would provide a valuable tool to assess the reliability of genomic information underlying regulatory decision-making.

2.2.3 Attribution of food vehicles through genomic surveillance

The advent of genomic typing augurs well for the creation of highly refined databases of bacterial isolates from various sources (foods, production facilities, farms, environmental and clinical strains) providing high-resolution characterization of individual strains with established linkages to their geographic and temporal origins. Historically, the use of low-resolution typing approaches such as MLST profiles or serotypes has been valuable for the association of specific lineages with a given food type, production environment, or country [70, 71]. Initiatives such as the GenomeTrakr and the PulseNet WGS networks represent rich resources from which to draw valuable information linking isolates to their origin in the food production continuum [6, 38, 72]. For example, an analysis of *E. coli* O157:H7 identified SNVs associated with country of origin [73]. Similarly, an outbreak involving *S.* Bareilly in the United States was tracked to a food originating in India based on high-resolution SNV typing [74].

With the aid of bioinformatics tools, databases can be queried to identify genomic signatures that are overrepresented in particular head sources for bacterial isolates. For example, a study by Thépault et al. [75] identified 15 host-associated *C. jejuni* markers and demonstrated utility of these markers for identifying host association of strains with 80% accuracy. The ability to discern this type of information would be a tremendous boon for foodborne illness investigations: WGS data could be used to determine the "source signature" of clinical isolates, enabling a highly proactive approach in rapidly narrowing the field for the attribution of food vehicles. Regulatory food inspection agencies such as the CFIA would have an important role to play in such a scheme. Ongoing, extensive sampling plans will be required to ensure adequate representation of different food production elements, such as food types and geographic provenance. Given that most cases of foodborne illness occur sporadically, this approach would enable public health authorities to track the causes of a larger proportion of cases of foodborne illness. This would ultimately lead to a better understanding of foods commonly implicated in disease and the implementation of more effective interventions to reduce the burden of foodborne illness.

2.3 Is it dangerous? Rapid identification of virulence, antimicrobial resistance, and epidemiological markers through WGS

Genomic information is highly complex, and there are many knowledge gaps with respect to the significance of various marker genes to public health [76]. Nonetheless, there is a growing body of evidence linking certain well-defined gene markers to virulence characteristics of bacteria, for example, the role of intimin (coded by the *eae* gene) in the pathogenesis of STEC, epidemiological associations between certain serotype features and outbreaks of serious foodborne illness (e.g., *L. monocytogenes* serogroups 1/2a, 1/2b, and 4b, STEC serogroups O26, O45, O103, O111, O121, O145, and O157), and even the type of toxin secreted (e.g., Shiga toxin 2) and the attendant severity of illness [77, 78].

In the case of STEC, regulatory food testing programs currently define priority target strains as bearing markers for Shiga toxin genes and intimin, in addition to markers associated with a narrow family of O serogroups [2]. However, the question arises whether in the course of conducting routine monitoring of food inspection samples the occurrence of an isolate bearing markers for Shiga toxin and intimin, but none of the so-called priority serogroups would be actionable. There are varying subjective opinions on the matter, ranging from a narrow interpretation of test results in which only isolates bearing all the designated factors are considered hazardous to the more precautionary approach whereby any isolate bearing both Shiga toxin and intimin factors, regardless of O serogroup, constitutes a public health risk. There is also evidence suggesting that severity or likelihood of foodborne illness varies with Shiga toxin type and subtype (e.g., STEC strains possessing st2a tend to be more frequently implicated in cases of severe foodborne illness [79]) and that this should be a factor in determining the appropriate response to the presence of a food contaminant. These properties are readily discoverable through the analysis of WGS data. For instance, the Shiga toxin subtype can be reliably determined using the V-typer tool, which is an automated assembly-independent subtyping module that can be integrated in a bioinformatics pipeline for the analysis of foodborne STEC isolates [23]. Yet another possibility would be to define priority STEC on the basis of contemporary public health data (reviewed periodically) identifying STEC serogroups most frequently associated with illness in a given jurisdiction. The serogroup of an *E. coli* isolate can be determined using tools such as SeroTypeFinder [8] which can be freely accessed through the Center for Genomic Epidemiology website [80].

Such considerations raise problems for health risk assessment specialists who must interpret laboratory results (among other factors) to determine the degree of risk informing the course of regulatory interventions [76]. It is tempting to speculate that it may be possible to devise an objective scheme for rating the degree of hazard associated with a given isolate on the basis of genomic analyses. For instance, the public health and food inspection communities could agree on a list of key factors relevant to the characterization of a given pathogen (**Table 1**). For organisms such as *E. coli*, acquired virulence gene databases have been established, and isolates may be profiled using tools such as VirulenceFinder [7], accessible through the Center for Genomic Epidemiology website [80]. Since not all factors have the same impact, it should be possible to develop a weighted index approach in which each constituent factor determined by genomic analysis makes up a fraction of a final index value which is proportional to the degree of hazard. Such an index value (hazard characterization or HazChar Score), used in conjunction with

Key factors	Element	Relevance
Primary virulence	Toxin	Presence or absence
	Attachment and colonization	*eae*, enteroaggregative factors
	Pathogenicity	Pathogenesis mechanisms (e.g., hemolysin)
Severity modulator	Type	*st*1 vs. *st2*
	Subtype	$st2_a$ vs. $st2_f$
Accessory functions	Antibiotic resistance	Therapeutic impact
	Antimicrobial resistance	Sanitizer efficacy
	Biofilm formation	Persistence
	Pathogenicity islands	Signatures for novel pathogens
Epidemiological markers	Serotype	Outbreak vs. sporadic vs. nil association
	Phage type	Reservoirs, illness outbreaks
	Molecular type	PFGE/SNV cluster
Phylogenetic markers	Genus/species	Identity (e.g., *Salmonella, E. coli*)
	Family or group	STEC

[a]A list of key factors is developed for a given pathogen, and each element is assigned a weighted value based on its significance in human illness. Genomic analysis of a foodborne isolate by whole-genome sequencing with the application of bioinformatics tools to determine the presence of targeted features. The individual weighted values are summed giving the HazChar Score, which is then compared against a set of predetermined criteria to categorize the degree of risk.

Table 1.
Proposed concept for hazard characterization: HazChar Score[a].

numerical criteria derived from historical data, could form a basis for attributing the degree of hazard associated with a particular isolate, which in turn would enable an objective categorization of risk to inform the appropriate regulatory response.

The antimicrobial resistance profile of pathogenic bacteria, while not a virulence attribute per se, remains an important factor in the ultimate public health outcomes of foodborne illness events, since a significant fraction of the affected population (e.g., the elderly and the immunocompromised) may critically require antibiotic therapy to recover. Furthermore, antimicrobial use at sub-therapeutic levels for growth promotion in food animal production has been implicated in the development of antimicrobial resistance (AMR) in animals and humans [81, 82], though there is paucity of data to support this claim. Food testing laboratories can play an important role in contributing data on the occurrence of AMR bacteria to national and international surveillance initiatives seeking to understand the role of production practices in the emergence of these microorganisms. As an alternative to labor- and time-consuming phenotypic testing, AMR profiles can be predicted from WGS data through the identification of genetic markers by querying the subject genome using DNA sequence information deposited in curated AMR gene databases, such as well-cataloged AMR gene markers. A number of tools are currently available to predict AMR from bacterial WGS data (e.g., ResFinder [10, 83], SEAR [84], Resistance Gene Identifier [85], and ARMI [86]). These AMR marker prediction tools rely on curated international AMR gene databases such as CARD [85], ARDB [87], and ARG-ANNOT [88]. WGS-based methods for prediction of AMR phenotype have been shown to be highly accurate [86, 89–91].

3. Future applications

3.1 Deployment of ad hoc methods in support of outbreak investigations

Despite recent efforts of regulatory food safety agencies to implement test methods targeting defined serogroups of so-called priority STEC, the history of foodborne disease outbreaks is rife with examples of causative strains with unexpected characteristics (e.g., the 2011 German outbreak in which the etiologic agent belonged to serogroup O104, not a designated priority serogroup, and lacked the definitive virulence marker *eae* [21]), making it difficult to anticipate detection methods suiting all contingencies. Detection is further complicated by variability among non-O157 STEC strains in resistance to selective agents commonly used in enrichment culture techniques, hindering their recovery from foods bearing high levels of background microbiota [92–94]. Genomic information garnered from clinical bacterial isolates implicated in outbreaks of foodborne illness will be very useful in the customization of selective recovery and identification procedures to facilitate their detection in food samples during outbreak investigations [86].

The state of the art in WGS technology has reached the point where clinical isolates implicated in foodborne disease outbreaks are routinely sequenced in public health laboratories at an early stage during these events [38]. With the application of appropriate bioinformatics tools to analyze the ensuing data, it should be possible to develop customized strain-specific test methods that can be rapidly deployed to food testing labs conducting analyses in support of outbreak investigations. The availability of WGS information for these strains should make it possible to ascertain the presence of traits conferring resistance to antimicrobial agents such as antibiotics, quaternary ammonium compounds, and tellurite, suggesting an avenue for the formulation of customized selective enrichment media enabling recovery of specific outbreak strains [86]. This would be a particular advantage in instances where a food matrix (e.g., meats, sprouts, etc.) contains high levels of background microbiota, which might otherwise interfere with recovery of the target organism. Genomic AMR prediction tools can be used to discern the AMR marker profile of a strain of interest (e.g., outbreak strain) to identify an antibiotic resistance trait which can be exploited for customization of selective enrichment media favoring its recovery from samples with high background bacteria loads [86, 95]. In addition, WGS data can be analyzed using a pipeline such as SigSeekr [96] designed to identify DNA sequences associated with a particular strain for its rapid identification by PCR. By combining strain-specific selective enrichment and PCR detection tools, it should be possible to deploy custom recovery and identification tools for the efficient detection of STEC outbreak strains within the timeframe of an active investigation. The feasibility of such an approach has been demonstrated using laboratory STEC strains as models, with resistance to a variety of antibiotic classes used as the basis for their selective recovery against high backgrounds of commensal *E. coli* bacteria in ground beef samples [86].

3.2 Characterization of food microbiomes in support of improved method development

Metagenomic analysis of enrichment dynamics can be used to inform the development of improved methods for cultural enrichment of pathogens [97–99]. A practical approach for this is to selectively amplify hypervariable regions within the 16 s rDNA and to sequence amplicons using WGS technologies. Sequences are then mapped to databases to determine composition of microbial communities using bioinformatics tools such as QIIME [100] or mothur [101]. Samples from enrichment cultures can be used to evaluate growth of target pathogens relative to background food microbiota over time [97, 99]. Such studies can provide valuable insight into species that could potentially interfere with target pathogens that can be applied to the development of improved methodology.

A modern concept in the study of pathogenic bacteria is the emergence of novel pathogens among commensals in a given environment through the acquisition of virulence factors by horizontal gene transfers from other bacteria [102–104]. The evolutionary trail of the STEC family suggests a priori transformations of benign *E. coli* strains into virulent STEC having acquired exogenous DNA segments such as bacteriophage carrying Shiga toxin genes and pathogenicity islands harboring host colonization factors [105]. There is evidence that other food pathogens such as *L. monocytogenes* strains implicated in serious outbreaks of foodborne illness may have acquired enhanced virulence characteristics through horizontal gene transfer processes [106]. This is believed to occur on a relatively short time scale, perhaps on the order of weeks or months, making the emergence of novel pathogens in food production environments or animal reservoirs in near real time a significant possibility. Furthermore, food-acquired coinfections may arise in which two or more bacterial strains complement each another, for example, a toxigenic strain lacking adherence factors might colonize a host by cross-utilizing a factor secreted by another strain [107]. It may be possible to predict the probability of emergence of novel pathogens with enhanced virulence or antibiotic resistance characteristics in the food supply through periodic microbial metagenomic analyses to ascertain the presence of key indicators in the background microflora of food commodities (e.g., ground beef, trim), food manufacturing environments (e.g., floors, food contact surfaces), and animal reservoirs (e.g., cattle, poultry) [108, 109]. A weighted index approach much like that described for the HazChar Score above could be employed here, with possible inclusion of a more comprehensive catalog of known virulence, AMR, and other critical factors relevant to public health.

4. Conclusions

Modern food microbiology research has generated a critical understanding of the epidemiology, pathogenic mechanisms, virulence factors, and other salient characteristics of the major food pathogens. The convergence of expanded scientific knowledge and sophisticated technological capability create exciting new opportunities for the refinement of food microbiology testing programs to meet the needs of a comprehensive risk-based inspection approach. Advances in next-generation sequencing technologies have made it possible for investigators to carry out sequencing and processing of bacterial genomes within the time course of a typical foodborne illness outbreak investigation. It may reasonably be expected that in the near future, analysts will be moving from traditional DNA hybridization approaches (e.g., PCR and microarrays) toward rapid whole-genome sequencing allowing a much more comprehensive examination of the isolate at hand. This new approach will require broad access to leading-edge bioinformatics capability for analysis of complex genomics data in silico to ascertain the presence of key genetic markers (e.g., presence of virulence genes in bacterial pathogens, completeness and functionality of gene products, markers for molecular typing, etc.). The generation and analysis of WGS information requires the migration of large packets of information between laboratory sites involved in the exploitation of this information, remote computing sites, and internet databases for data manipulation and comparative analyses. There are many ways in which the high-tech needs of the future can be met, even for relatively small laboratories with low operating budgets.

Opportunities abound for food inspection, public health, and academic laboratories to pool their resources and serve one another in the common purpose of safeguarding citizens from preventable food-acquired illness.

Acknowledgements

The authors thank Paul Manninger, Mylène Deschênes, and Martine Dixon for providing laboratory support throughout many years in developing the food pathogen genomics program at the Canadian Food Inspection Agency and Andrew Low for providing bioinformatics support and for critical review of this manuscript.

Author details

Catherine D. Carrillo, Adam Koziol, Neil Vary and Burton W. Blais*
Research and Development, Ottawa Laboratory (Carling), Canadian Food Inspection Agency, Ottawa, Ontario, Canada

*Address all correspondence to: burton.blais@canada.ca

References

[1] Blais BW, Gauthier M, Deschênes M, Huszczynski G. Polyester cloth-based hybridization array system for identification of enterohemorrhagic *Escherichia coli* serogroups O26, O45, O103, O111, O121, O145, and O157. Journal of Food Protection. 2012;**75**:1691-1697. DOI: 10.4315/0362-028X.JFP-12-116

[2] Blais BW, Gauthier M, Deschenes M, Huszczynski G. Characterization of verotoxigenic *Escherichia coli* O157:H7 colonies by polymerase chain reaction (PCR) and cloth-based hybridization array system (CHAS) (MFLP-22). In: Compendium of Analytical Methods, Laboratory Procedures for the Microbiological Analysis of Foods. Vol. 3. Ottawa, Canada: Health Canada; 2013. https://www.canada.ca/en/health-canada/services/food-nutrition/research-programs-analytical-methods/analytical-methods/compendium-methods.html [Accessed: February 20, 2019]

[3] Blais BW, Martinez A, Gill A, McIlwham S, Mohajer S, Gauthier M. Isolation and identification of priority verotoxigenic *Escherichia coli* (VTEC) in meat and vegetable products (MFLP-52). In: Compendium of Methods, Laboratory Procedures for the Microbiological Analysis of Foods. Vol. 3. Ottawa, Canada: Health Canada; 2014. Available from: https://www.canada.ca/en/health-canada/services/food-nutrition/ research-programs-analytical-methods/analytical-methods/ compendium-methods.html [Accessed: February 20, 2019]

[4] Huszczynski G, Gauthier M, Mohajer S, Gill A, Blais B. Method for the detection of priority Shiga toxin-producing *Escherichia coli* in beef trim. Journal of Food Protection. 2013;**76**:1689-1696. DOI: 10.4315/0362-028X.JFP-13-059

[5] Lambert D, Carrillo CD, Koziol AG, Manninger P, Blais BW. GeneSippr: A rapid whole-genome approach for the identification and characterization of foodborne pathogens such as priority Shiga toxigenic *Escherichia coli*. PLoS One. 2015;**10**:e0122928. DOI: 10.1371/journal.pone.0122928

[6] Allard MW, Strain E, Melka D, Bunning K, Musser SM, Brown EW, et al. Practical value of food pathogen traceability through building a whole-genome sequencing network and database. Journal of Clinical Microbiology. 2016;**54**:1975-1983. DOI: 10.1128/JCM.00081-16

[7] Joensen KG, Scheutz F, Lund O, Hasman H, Kaas RS, Nielsen EM, et al. Real-time whole-genome sequencing for routine typing, surveillance, and outbreak detection of verotoxigenic *Escherichia coli*. Journal of Clinical Microbiology. 2014;**52**:1501-1510. DOI: 10.1128/JCM.03617-13

[8] Joensen KG, Tetzschner AMM, Iguchi A, Aarestrup FM, Scheutz F. Rapid and easy *in silico* serotyping of *Escherichia coli* isolates by use of whole-genome sequencing data. Journal of Clinical Microbiology. 2015;**53**:2410-2426. DOI: 10.1128/JCM.00008-15

[9] Yoshida CE, Kruczkiewicz P, Laing CR, Lingohr EJ, Gannon VPJ, Nash JHE, et al. The *Salmonella* In Silico Typing Resource (SISTR): An open web-accessible tool for rapidly typing and subtyping draft *Salmonella* genome assemblies. PLoS One. 2016;**11**:e0147101. DOI: 10.1371/journal.pone.0147101

[10] Kleinheinz KA, Joensen KG, Larsen MV. Applying the ResFinder and VirulenceFinder web-services for easy identification of acquired antibiotic resistance and *E. coli* virulence genes in bacteriophage and prophage

nucleotide sequences. Bacteriophage. 2014;**4**:e27943. DOI: 10.4161/bact.27943

[11] Ronholm J, Nasheri N, Petronella N, Pagotto F. Navigating microbiological food safety in the era of whole-genome sequencing. Clinical Microbiology Reviews. 2016;**29**:837-857. DOI: 10.1128/CMR.00056-16

[12] Sharapov UM, Wendel AM, Davis JP, Keene WE, Farrar J, Sodha S, et al. Multistate outbreak of *Escherichia coli* O157:H7 infections associated with consumption of fresh spinach: United States, 2006. Journal of Food Protection. 2016;**79**:2024-2030. DOI: 10.4315/0362-028X.JFP-15-556

[13] Berenger BM, Berry C, Peterson T, Fach P, Delannoy S, Li V, et al. The utility of multiple molecular methods including whole genome sequencing as tools to differentiate *Escherichia coli* O157:H7 outbreaks. Eurosurveillance. 2015;**20**:30073. DOI: 10.2807/1560-7917.ES.2015.20.47.30073

[14] Seys SA, Sampedro F, Hedberg CW. Assessment of Shiga toxin–producing *Escherichia coli* O157 illnesses prevented by recalls of beef products. Foodborne Pathogens and Disease. 2015;**12**:800-805. DOI: 10.1089/fpd.2015.1968

[15] Microbiological Methods Committee. Isolation of *Escherichia coli* O157:H7/NM from foods and environmental surface samples (MFHPB-10). In: Compend. Anal Methods. Ottawa, Canada: Health Canada. Vol. 2. Ottawa, Canada: Health Canada; 2017. Available from: https://www.canada.ca/en/health-canada/services/food-nutrition/ research-programs-analytical-methods/analytical-methods/compendium-methods.html [Accessed: February 20, 2019]

[16] USDA-FSIS. Detection, isolation and identification of top seven Shiga toxin-producing *Escherichia coli* (STECs) from meat products and carcass and environmental sponges. United States Department of Agriculture, Athens, GA, 2019. Available from: https://www.fsis.usda.gov/wps/wcm/connect/fsis-content/internet/main/topics/science/laboratories-and-procedures/guidebooks-and-methods/microbiology-laboratory-guidebook/microbiology-laboratory-guidebook [Accessed April 18, 2019]

[17] Martinez-Perez A, Blais BW. Cloth-based hybridization array system for the identification of *Escherichia coli* O157:H7. Food Control. 2010;**21**:1354-1359. DOI: 10.1016/j.foodcont.2010.04.009

[18] Health Canada. The Compendium of Analytical Methods. n.d. Available from: https://www.canada.ca/en/health-canada/services/food-nutrition/research-programs-analytical-methods/analytical-methods/compendium-methods.html [Accessed: February 20, 2019]

[19] Catford A, Kouamé V, Martinez-Perez A, Gill A, Buenaventura E, Couture H, et al. Risk profile on non-O157 verotoxin-producing *Escherichia coli* in produce, beef, milk and dairy products in Canada. International Food Risk Analysis Journal. 2014;**4**:1-25. DOI: 10.5772/59208

[20] EFSA Panel on Biological Hazards (BIOHAZ). Scientific opinion on VTEC-seropathotype and scientific criteria regarding pathogenicity assessment. EFSA Journal. 2013;**11**:3138. DOI: 10.2903/j.efsa.2013.3138

[21] Burger R. EHEC O104:H4 in Germany 2011: Large Outbreak of Bloody Diarrhea and Haemolytic Uraemic Syndrome by Shiga Toxin-producing E. coli via Contaminated Food. In: Institute of Medicine (US). Improving Food Safety Through a One Health Approach: Workshop Summary. Washington DC: National Academies Press (US); 2012.

Available from: https://www.ncbi.nlm.nih.gov/books/NBK114499/[Accessed February 20, 2019]

[22] Frank C, Werber D, Cramer JP, Askar M, Faber M, an der Heiden M, et al. Epidemic profile of Shiga-toxin–producing *Escherichia coli* O104:H4 outbreak in Germany. The New England Journal of Medicine. 2011;**365**:1771-1780. DOI: 10.1056/NEJMoa1106483

[23] Carrillo CD, Koziol AG, Mathews A, Goji N, Lambert D, Huszczynski G, et al. Comparative evaluation of genomic and laboratory approaches for determination of Shiga toxin subtypes in *Escherichia coli*. Journal of Food Protection. 2016;**79**:2078-2085. DOI: 10.4315/0362-028X.JFP-16-228

[24] Lambert D, Pightling A, Griffiths E, Van Domselaar G, Evans P, Berthelet S, et al. Baseline practices for the application of genomic data supporting regulatory food safety. Journal of AOAC International. 2017;**100**:721-731. DOI: 10.5740/jaoacint.16-0269

[25] Low AJ, Koziol AG, Manninger PA, Blais BW, Carrillo CD. ConFindr: Rapid detection of intraspecies and cross-species contamination in bacterial whole-genome sequence data. 2019;7:e27499v1. DOI: 10.7287/peerj.preprints.27499v1

[26] Angers-Loustau A, Petrillo M, Bengtsson-Palme J, Berendonk T, Blais B, Chan K-G, et al. The challenges of designing a benchmark strategy for bioinformatics pipelines in the identification of antimicrobial resistance determinants using next generation sequencing technologies. F1000 Research. 2018;**7**:459. DOI: 10.12688/f1000research.14509.2

[27] Ribot EM, Hise KB. Future challenges for tracking foodborne diseases: PulseNet, a 20-year-old US surveillance system for foodborne diseases, is expanding both globally and technologically. EMBO Reports. 2016;**17**:1499-1505. DOI: 10.15252/embr.201643128

[28] Swaminathan B, Barrett TJ, Hunter SB, Tauxe RV, CDC PulseNet Task Force. PulseNet: The molecular subtyping network for foodborne bacterial disease surveillance, United States. Emerging Infectious Diseases. 2001;7:382-389. DOI: 10.3201/eid0703.010303

[29] Taboada EN, Clark CG, Sproston EL, Carrillo CD. Current methods for molecular typing of *Campylobacter* species. Journal of Microbiological Methods. 2013;**95**:24-31. DOI: 10.1016/j.mimet.2013.07.007

[30] Herikstad H, Motarjemi Y, Tauxe RV. *Salmonella* surveillance: A global survey of public health serotyping. Epidemiology and Infection. 2002;**129**:1-8

[31] Penner JL, Hennessy JN. Passive hemagglutination technique for serotyping *Campylobacter fetus* subsp. *jejuni* on the basis of soluble heat-stable antigens. Journal of Clinical Microbiology. 1980;**12**:732-737

[32] Evans DJ, Evans DG. Classification of pathogenic *Escherichia coli* according to serotype and the production of virulence factors, with special reference to colonization-factor antigens. Reviews of Infectious Diseases. 1983;**5**(Suppl 4):S692-S701

[33] Hickman-Brenner FW, Stubbs AD, Farmer JJ. Phage typing of *Salmonella* enteritidis in the United States. Journal of Clinical Microbiology. 1991;**29**:2817-2823

[34] Maiden MCJ. Multilocus sequence typing of bacteria. Annual Review of Microbiology. 2006;**60**:561-588. DOI: 10.1146/annurev.micro.59.030804.121325

[35] Maiden MCJ, Bygraves JA, Feil E, Morelli G, Russell JE, Urwin R, et al. Multilocus sequence typing: A portable approach to the identification of clones within populations of pathogenic microorganisms. Proceedings of the National Academy of Sciences of the United States of America. 1998;**95**:3140-3145

[36] Schjørring S, Niskanen T, Torpdahl M, Björkman JT, Nielsen EM. Evaluation of molecular typing of foodborne pathogens in European reference laboratories from 2012 to 2013. Euro Surveillance. 2016;**21**:pii=30429. DOI: 10.2807/1560-7917.ES.2016.21.50.30429

[37] Barrett TJ, Lior H, Green JH, Khakhria R, Wells JG, Bell BP, et al. Laboratory investigation of a multistate food-borne outbreak of *Escherichia coli* O157:H7 by using pulsed-field gel electrophoresis and phage typing. Journal of Clinical Microbiology. 1994;**32**:3013-3017

[38] Nadon C, Van Walle I, Gerner-Smidt P, Campos J, Chinen I, Concepcion-Acevedo J, et al. PulseNet international: Vision for the implementation of whole genome sequencing (WGS) for global food-borne disease surveillance. Eurosurveillance. 2017;**22**:pii=30544. DOI: 10.2807/1560-7917.ES.2017.22.23.30544

[39] Grant K, Jenkins C, Arnold C, Green J, Zambon M. Implementing Pathogen Genomics: A Case Study. Public Health England. 2018. Available from: https://www.gov.uk/government/publications/implementing-pathogen-genomics-a-case-study [Accessed February 23, 2019]

[40] Deng X, Desai PT, den Bakker HC, Mikoleit M, Tolar B, Trees E, et al. Genomic epidemiology of *Salmonella enterica* serotype Enteritidis based on population structure of prevalent lineages. Emerging Infectious Diseases. 2014;**20**:1481-1489. DOI: 10.3201/eid2009.131095

[41] Jagadeesan B, Gerner-Smidt P, Allard MW, Leuillet S, Winkler A, Xiao Y, et al. The use of next generation sequencing for improving food safety: Translation into practice. Food Microbiology. 2019;**79**:96-115. DOI: 10.1016/j.fm.2018.11.005

[42] Petkau A, Mabon P, Sieffert C, Knox NC, Cabral J, Iskander M, et al. SNVPhyl: A single nucleotide variant phylogenomics pipeline for microbial genomic epidemiology. Microbial Genomics. 2017;**3**:e000116. DOI: 10.1099/mgen.0.000116

[43] Markell JA, Koziol AG, Lambert D. Draft genome sequence of *Escherichia coli* O157:H7 ATCC 35150 and a nalidixic acid-resistant mutant derivative. Genome Announcements. 2015;**3**:e00734-15. DOI: 10.1128/genomeA.00734-15

[44] Maiden MCJ, Jansen van Rensburg MJ, Bray JE, Earle SG, Ford SA, Jolley KA, et al. MLST revisited: The gene-by-gene approach to bacterial genomics. Nature Reviews. Microbiology. 2013;**11**:728-736. DOI: 10.1038/nrmicro3093

[45] Carrillo CD, Kruczkiewicz P, Mutschall S, Tudor A, Clark C, Taboada EN. A framework for assessing the concordance of molecular typing methods and the true strain phylogeny of *Campylobacter jejuni* and *C. coli* using draft genome sequence data. Frontiers in Cellular and Infection Microbiology. 2012;**2**:57. DOI: 10.3389/fcimb.2012.00057

[46] Jolley KA, Bliss CM, Bennett JS, Bratcher HB, Brehony C, Colles FM, et al. Ribosomal multilocus sequence typing: Universal characterization of bacteria from domain to strain. Microbiology. 2012;**158**:1005-1015. DOI: 10.1099/mic.0.055459-0

[47] Chen Y, Luo Y, Carleton H, Timme R, Melka D, Muruvanda T, et al. Whole genome and core genome multilocus sequence typing and single nucleotide polymorphism analyses of *Listeria monocytogenes* associated with an outbreak linked to cheese, United States, 2013. Applied and Environmental Microbiology. 2017;**83**:pii: e00633-17. DOI: 10.1128/AEM.00633-17

[48] Gilmour MW, Graham M, Reimer A, Van Domselaar G. Public health genomics and the new molecular epidemiology of bacterial pathogens. Public Health Genomics. 2013;**16**:25-30. DOI: 10.1159/000342709

[49] LeClerc JE, Li B, Payne WL, Cebula TA. High mutation frequencies among *Escherichia coli* and *Salmonella* pathogens. Science. 1996;**274**:1208-1211. DOI: 10.1126/science.274.5290.1208

[50] Kozyreva VK, Ilina EN, Malakhova MV, Carattoli A, Azizov IS, Tapalski DV, et al. Long-term dissemination of CTX-M-5-producing hypermutable *Salmonella enterica* serovar typhimurium sequence type 328 strains in Russia, Belarus, and Kazakhstan. Antimicrobial Agents and Chemotherapy. 2014;**58**:5202-5210. DOI: 10.1128/AAC.02506-14

[51] Pope CF, O'Sullivan DM, McHugh TD, Gillespie SH. A practical guide to measuring mutation rates in antibiotic resistance. Antimicrobial Agents and Chemotherapy. 2008;**52**:1209-1214. DOI: 10.1128/AAC.01152-07

[52] Eliopoulos GM, Blázquez J. Hypermutation as a factor contributing to the acquisition of antimicrobial resistance. Clinical Infectious Diseases. 2003;**37**:1201-1209. DOI: 10.1086/378810

[53] Swings T, Van den Bergh B, Wuyts S, Oeyen E, Voordeckers K, Verstrepen KJ, et al. Adaptive tuning of mutation rates allows fast response to lethal stress in *Escherichia coli*. eLife. 2017;**6**:e22939. DOI: 10.7554/eLife.22939

[54] Leong D, Alvarez-Ordóñez A, Jordan K. Monitoring occurrence and persistence of *Listeria monocytogenes* in foods and food processing environments in the Republic of Ireland. Frontiers in Microbiology. 2014;**5**:436. DOI: 10.3389/fmicb.2014.00436

[55] Nastasijevic I, Milanov D, Velebit B, Djordjevic V, Swift C, Painset A, et al. Tracking of *Listeria monocytogenes* in meat establishment using whole genome sequencing as a food safety management tool: A proof of concept. International Journal of Food Microbiology. 2017;**257**:157-164. DOI: 10.1016/j.ijfoodmicro.2017.06.015

[56] Malley TJV, Butts J, Wiedmann M. Seek and destroy process: *Listeria monocytogenes* process controls in the ready-to-eat meat and poultry industry. Journal of Food Protection. 2015;**78**:436-445. DOI: 10.4315/0362-028X.JFP-13-507

[57] Thomas MK, Murray R, Flockhart L, Pintar K, Fazil A, Nesbitt A, et al. Estimates of foodborne illness-related hospitalizations and deaths in Canada for 30 specified pathogens and unspecified agents. Foodborne Pathogens and Disease. 2015;**12**:820-827. DOI: 10.1089/fpd.2015.1966

[58] Government of Canada. Report of the Independent Investigator into the 2008 listeriosis outbreak 2009. Available from: http://publications.gc.ca/site/eng/361474/publication.html [Accessed: February 18, 2019]

[59] Cherifi T, Carrillo C, Lambert D, Miniaï I, Quessy S, Larivière-Gauthier G, et al. Genomic characterization of *Listeria monocytogenes* isolates

reveals that their persistence in a pig slaughterhouse is linked to the presence of benzalkonium chloride resistance genes. BMC Microbiology. 2018;**18**:220. DOI: 10.1186/s12866-018-1363-9

[60] Martínez-Suárez JV, Ortiz S, López-Alonso V. Potential impact of the resistance to quaternary ammonium disinfectants on the persistence of *Listeria monocytogenes* in food processing environments. Frontiers in Microbiology. 2016;**7**:638. DOI: 10.3389/fmicb.2016.00638

[61] Yu T, Jiang X, Zhang Y, Ji S, Gao W, Shi L. Effect of benzalkonium chloride adaptation on sensitivity to antimicrobial agents and tolerance to environmental stresses in *Listeria monocytogenes*. Frontiers in Microbiology. 2018;**9**:2906. DOI: 10.3389/fmicb.2018.02906

[62] Elhanafi D, Dutta V, Kathariou S. Genetic characterization of plasmid-associated benzalkonium chloride resistance determinants in a *Listeria monocytogenes* strain from the 1998-1999 outbreak. Applied and Environmental Microbiology. 2010;**76**:8231-8238. DOI: 10.1128/AEM.02056-10

[63] Kovacevic J, Ziegler J, Wałecka-Zacharska E, Reimer A, Kitts DD, Gilmour MW. Tolerance of *Listeria monocytogenes* to quaternary ammonium sanitizers is mediated by a novel efflux pump encoded by *emrE*. Applied and Environmental Microbiology. 2016;**82**:939-953. DOI: 10.1128/AEM.03741-15

[64] Franz E, Gras LM, Dallman T. Significance of whole genome sequencing for surveillance, source attribution and microbial risk assessment of foodborne pathogens. Current Opinion in Food Science. 2016;**8**:74-79. DOI: 10.1016/j.cofs.2016.04.004

[65] Schjørring S, Lassen SG, Jensen T, Moura A, Kjeldgaard JS, Müller L, et al. Cross-border outbreak of listeriosis caused by cold-smoked salmon, revealed by integrated surveillance and whole genome sequencing (WGS), Denmark and France, 2015 to 2017. Eurosurveillance. 2017;**22**:17-00762. DOI: 10.2807/1560-7917.ES.2017.22.50.17-00762

[66] Lienau EK, Strain E, Wang C, Zheng J, Ottesen AR, Keys CE, et al. Identification of a salmonellosis outbreak by means of molecular sequencing. The New England Journal of Medicine. 2011;**364**:981-982. DOI: 10.1056/NEJMc1100443

[67] Rantsiou K, Kathariou S, Winkler A, Skandamis P, Saint-Cyr MJ, Rouzeau-Szynalski K, et al. Next generation microbiological risk assessment: Opportunities of whole genome sequencing (WGS) for foodborne pathogen surveillance, source tracking and risk assessment. International Journal of Food Microbiology. 2018;**287**:3-9. DOI: 10.1016/j.ijfoodmicro.2017.11.007

[68] National Research Council (US) Committee on DNA Forensic Science: An Update. The Evaluation of Forensic DNA Evidence.5. Statistical Issues. Washington DC: National Academies Press (US); 1996. Available from: https://www.ncbi.nlm.nih.gov/books/NBK232615/ [Accessed February 24 2019]

[69] Wilson MR, Allard MW, Brown EW. The forensic analysis of foodborne bacterial pathogens in the age of whole-genome sequencing. Cladistics. 2013;**29**:449-461. DOI: 10.1111/cla.12012

[70] Rosner BM, Schielke A, Didelot X, Kops F, Breidenbach J, Willrich N, et al. A combined case-control and molecular source attribution study of human *Campylobacter* infections

in Germany, 2011-2014. Scientific Reports. 2017;**7**:5139. DOI: 10.1038/s41598-017-05227-x

[71] Pires SM, Vieira AR, Hald T, Cole D. Source attribution of human salmonellosis: An overview of methods and estimates. Foodborne Pathogens and Disease. 2014;**11**:667-676. DOI: 10.1089/fpd.2014.1744

[72] Yachison CA, Yoshida C, Robertson J, Nash JHE, Kruczkiewicz P, Taboada EN, et al. The validation and implications of using whole genome sequencing as a replacement for traditional serotyping for a National *Salmonella* Reference Laboratory. Frontiers in Microbiology. 2017;**8**:1044. DOI: 10.3389/fmicb.2017.01044

[73] Mellor GE, Fegan N, Gobius KS, Smith HV, Jennison AV, D'Astek BA, et al. Geographically distinct *Escherichia coli* O157 isolates differ by lineage, Shiga toxin genotype, and total Shiga toxin production. Journal of Clinical Microbiology. 2015;**53**:579-586. DOI: 10.1128/JCM.01532-14

[74] Hoffmann M, Luo Y, Monday SR, Gonzalez-Escalona N, Ottesen AR, Muruvanda T, et al. Tracing origins of the *Salmonella* Bareilly Strain causing a food-borne outbreak in the United States. The Journal of Infectious Diseases. 2016;**213**:502-508. DOI: 10.1093/infdis/jiv297

[75] Thépault A, Méric G, Rivoal K, Pascoe B, Mageiros L, Touzain F, et al. Genome-wide identification of host-segregating epidemiological markers for source attribution in *Campylobacter jejuni*. Applied and Environmental Microbiology. 2017;**83**. DOI: 10.1128/AEM.03085-16

[76] Cocolin L, Membré J-M, Zwietering MH. Editorial: Integration of omics into MRA. International Journal of Food Microbiology. 2018;**287**:1-2. DOI: 10.1016/j.ijfoodmicro.2017.11.006

[77] Farber JM, Peterkin PI. *Listeria monocytogenes*, a food-borne pathogen. Microbiological Reviews. 1991;**55**:476-511

[78] de Boer RF, Ferdous M, Ott A, Scheper HR, Wisselink GJ, Heck ME, et al. Assessing the public health risk of Shiga toxin-producing *Escherichia coli* by use of a rapid diagnostic screening algorithm. Journal of Clinical Microbiology. 2015;**53**:1588-1598. DOI: 10.1128/JCM.03590-14

[79] Ashton PM, Perry N, Ellis R, Petrovska L, Wain J, Grant KA, et al. Insight into Shiga toxin genes encoded by *Escherichia coli* O157 from whole genome sequencing. PeerJ. 2015;**3**:e739. DOI: 10.7717/peerj.739

[80] Center for Genomic Epidemiology. n.d. Available from: http://www.genomicepidemiology.org/ [Accessed: February 20, 2019]

[81] Dutil L, Irwin R, Finley R, Ng LK, Avery B, Boerlin P, et al. Ceftiofur resistance in *Salmonella enterica* serovar Heidelberg from chicken meat and humans, Canada. Emerging Infectious Diseases. 2010;**16**:48-54. DOI: 10.3201/eid1601.090729

[82] Tang KL, Caffrey NP, Nóbrega DB, Cork SC, Ronksley PE, Barkema HW, et al. Restricting the use of antibiotics in food-producing animals and its associations with antibiotic resistance in food-producing animals and human beings: A systematic review and meta-analysis. Lancet Planetary Health. 2017;**1**:e316-e327. DOI: 10.1016/S2542-5196(17)30141-9

[83] Zankari E, Hasman H, Cosentino S, Vestergaard M, Rasmussen S, Lund O, et al. Identification of acquired antimicrobial resistance genes. The Journal of Antimicrobial Chemotherapy. 2012;**67**:2640-2644. DOI: 10.1093/jac/dks261

[84] Rowe W, Baker KS, Verner-Jeffreys D, Baker-Austin C, Ryan JJ, Maskell D, et al. Search engine for antimicrobial resistance: A cloud compatible pipeline and web interface for rapidly detecting antimicrobial resistance genes directly from sequence data. PLoS One. 2015;**10**:e0133492. DOI: 10.1371/journal.pone.0133492

[85] McArthur AG, Waglechner N, Nizam F, Yan A, Azad MA, Baylay AJ, et al. The comprehensive antibiotic resistance database. Antimicrobial Agents and Chemotherapy. 2013;**57**:3348-3357. DOI: 10.1128/AAC.00419-13

[86] Knowles M, Stinson S, Lambert D, Carrillo C, Koziol A, Gauthier M, et al. Genomic tools for customized recovery and detection of foodborne Shiga toxigenic *Escherichia coli*. Journal of Food Protection. 2016;**79**: 2066-2077. DOI: 10.4315/0362-028X.JFP-16-220

[87] Liu B, Pop M. ARDB-antibiotic resistance genes database. Nucleic Acids Research. 2009;**37**:D443-D447. DOI: 10.1093/nar/gkn656

[88] Gupta SK, Padmanabhan BR, Diene SM, Lopez-Rojas R, Kempf M, Landraud L, et al. ARG-ANNOT, a new bioinformatic tool to discover antibiotic resistance genes in bacterial genomes. Antimicrobial Agents and Chemotherapy. 2014;**58**:212-220. DOI: 10.1128/AAC.01310-13

[89] Tyson GH, McDermott PF, Li C, Chen Y, Tadesse DA, Mukherjee S, et al. WGS accurately predicts antimicrobial resistance in *Escherichia coli*. The Journal of Antimicrobial Chemotherapy. 2015;**70**:2763-2769. DOI: 10.1093/jac/dkv186

[90] McDermott PF, Tyson GH, Kabera C, Chen Y, Li C, Folster JP, et al. Whole-genome sequencing for detecting antimicrobial resistance in nontyphoidal *Salmonella*. Antimicrobial Agents and Chemotherapy. 2016;**60**:5515-5520. DOI: 10.1128/AAC.01030-16

[91] Zhao S, Tyson GH, Chen Y, Li C, Mukherjee S, Young S, et al. Whole genome sequencing analysis accurately predicts antimicrobial resistance phenotypes in *Campylobacter*. Applied and Environmental Microbiology. 2015;**82**:459-466. DOI:10.1128/AEM.02873-15

[92] Gill A, Huszczynski G, Gauthier M, Blais B. Evaluation of eight agar media for the isolation of Shiga toxin-producing *Escherichia coli*. Journal of Microbiological Methods. 2014;**96**:6-11. DOI: 10.1016/j.mimet.2013.10.022

[93] Gill A, Martinez-Perez A, McIlwham S, Blais B. Development of a method for the detection of Verotoxin-producing *Escherichia coli* in food. Journal of Food Protection. 2012;**75**: 827-837. DOI: 10.4315/0362-028X.JFP-11-395

[94] Vimont A, Delignette-Muller M-L, Vernozy-Rozand C. Supplementation of enrichment broths by novobiocin for detecting Shiga toxin-producing *Escherichia coli* from food: A controversial use. Letters in Applied Microbiology. 2007;**44**:326-331. DOI: 10.1111/j.1472-765X.2006.02059.x

[95] Blais BW, Tapp K, Dixon M, Carrillo CD. Genomically informed strain-specific recovery of Shiga toxin-producing *Escherichia coli* during foodborne illness outbreak investigations. Journal of Food Protection. 2019;**82**:39-44. DOI: 10.4315/0362-028X.JFP-18-340

[96] Knowles M, Lambert D, Huszczynski G, Gauthier M, Blais BW. PCR for the specific selection of an *Escherichia coli* O157:H7 laboratory control strain. Journal of Food

Protection. 2015;**78**:1738-1744. DOI: 10.4315/0362-028X.JFP-15-147

[97] Margot H, Tasara T, Zwietering MH, Joosten H, Stephan R. Effects of different media on the enrichment of low numbers of Shiga toxin-producing *Escherichia coli* in mung bean sprouts and on the development of the sprout microbiome. International Journal of Food Microbiology. 2016;**232**:26-34. DOI: 10.1016/j.ijfoodmicro.2016.05.005

[98] Jarvis KG, Daquigan N, White JR, Morin PM, Howard LM, Manetas JE, et al. Microbiomes associated with foods from plant and animal sources. Frontiers in Microbiology. 2018;**9**:2540. DOI: 10.3389/fmicb.2018.02540

[99] Ottesen A, Ramachandran P, Reed E, White JR, Hasan N, Subramanian P, et al. Enrichment dynamics of *Listeria monocytogenes* and the associated microbiome from naturally contaminated ice cream linked to a listeriosis outbreak. BMC Microbiology. 2016;**16**:275. DOI: 10.1186/s12866-016-0894-1

[100] Caporaso JG, Kuczynski J, Stombaugh J, Bittinger K, Bushman FD, Costello EK, et al. QIIME allows analysis of high-throughput community sequencing data. Nature Methods. 2010;**7**:335-336. DOI: 10.1038/nmeth.f.303

[101] Schloss PD, Westcott SL, Ryabin T, Hall JR, Hartmann M, Hollister EB, et al. Introducing mothur: Open-source, platform-independent, community-supported software for describing and comparing microbial communities. Applied and Environmental Microbiology. 2009;**75**:7537-7541. DOI: 10.1128/AEM.01541-09

[102] Morschhäuser J, Köhler G, Ziebuhr W, Blum-Oehler G, Dobrindt U, Hacker J. Evolution of microbial pathogens. Philosophical Transactions of the Royal Society of London. Series B, Biological Sciences. 2000;**355**:695-704. DOI: 10.1098/rstb.2000.0609

[103] Iraola G, Pérez R, Naya H, Paolicchi F, Pastor E, Valenzuela S, et al. Genomic evidence for the emergence and evolution of pathogenicity and niche preferences in the genus *Campylobacter*. Genome Biology and Evolution. 2014;**6**:2392-2405. DOI: 10.1093/gbe/evu195

[104] Wirth T, Falush D, Lan R, Colles F, Mensa P, Wieler LH, et al. Sex and virulence in *Escherichia coli*: An evolutionary perspective. Molecular Microbiology. 2006;**60**:1136-1151. DOI: 10.1111/j.1365-2958.2006.05172.x

[105] Lacher DW. The evolutionary model of *Escherichia coli* O157:H7. In: Walk S, Feng P, editors. Population Genetics of Bacteria. Washington, DC: ASM Press; 2011:227-239. DOI: 10.1128/9781555817114.ch13

[106] Kelly BG, Vespermann A, Bolton DJ. Horizontal gene transfer of virulence determinants in selected bacterial foodborne pathogens. Food and Chemical Toxicology: An International Journal Published for the British Industrial Biological Research Association. 2009;**47**:969-977. DOI: 10.1016/j.fct.2008.02.007

[107] Gilmour MW, Tabor H, Wang G, Clark CG, Tracz DM, Olson AB, et al. Isolation and genetic characterization of a coinfection of non-O157 Shiga toxin-producing *Escherichia coli*. Journal of Clinical Microbiology. 2007;**45**: 3771-3773. DOI: 10.1128/JCM.01125-07

[108] Oniciuc EA, Likotrafiti E, Alvarez-Molina A, Prieto M, Santos JA, Alvarez-Ordóñez A. The present and future of whole genome sequencing (WGS) and whole metagenome sequencing (WMS) for surveillance of antimicrobial resistant microorganisms and antimicrobial resistance genes across the food chain. Genes. 2018;**9**:268. DOI: 10.3390/genes9050268

[109] Auffret MD, Dewhurst RJ, Duthie C-A, Rooke JA, John Wallace R, Freeman TC, et al. The rumen microbiome as a reservoir of antimicrobial resistance and pathogenicity genes is directly affected by diet in beef cattle. Microbiome. 2017;5:159. DOI: 10.1186/s40168-017-0378-z